Mental Disability and Rehabilitation SOURCEBOOK

FIRST EDITION

Disability Series

Mental Disability and Rehabilitation SOURCEBOOK

FIRST EDITION

Basic Consumer Health Information about Different Types of Mental and Psychotic Disorders, Impact of Mental Disability on Personal, Social, and Economic Well-Being, Treatment and Rehabilitation with Psychotherapies, as well as Crisis Assistance, Suicide Prevention, and Rights and Benefits of People with Mental Disabilities, and Tips for Mental Disabilities Support

Along with Facts about Rehabilitative and Integrated Care and Resources for Additional Information and Services

OMNIGRAPHICS
615 Griswold St., Ste. 520, Detroit, MI 48226

* * *

OMNIGRAPHICS
Angela L. Williams, *Managing Editor*

* * *

ISBN 978-0-7808-1766-1
E-ISBN 978-0-7808-1771-5

Library of Congress Cataloging-in-Publication Data

Names: Williams, Angela, 1963- editor.

Title: Mental disability and rehabilitation sourcebook / Angela L. Williams.

Description: First edition. | Detroit : Omnigraphics, Inc., 2019. | Series: Disability special series | Summary: "Offers basic consumer health information about barriers faced by people with mental disabilities, causes for disturbances of emotional equilibrium, mental-health services, and rehabilitation with brain stimulation therapies, as well as crisis assistance, social security disability insurance, and compensation. A directory of organizations for people with disabilities."--Provided by publisher"-- Provided by publisher.

Identifiers: LCCN 2019034482 (print) | LCCN 2019034483 (ebook) | ISBN 9780780817661 (library binding) | ISBN 9780780817715 (ebook)

Subjects: LCSH: Mentally ill--Rehabilitation--Handbooks, manuals, etc.

Classification: LCC RC439.5.M46 2019 (print) | LCC RC439.5 (ebook) | DDC 362.2--dc23

LC record available at https://lccn.loc.gov/2019034482

LC ebook record available at https://lccn.loc.gov/2019034483

Printed in the United States

Table of Contents

PART 3: Recovery, Rehabilitation, and Caregiving

PART 4: Protections, Rights, and Benefits

Preface

ABOUT THIS BOOK

Mental disability is an impairment or long-term loss of mental function. It affects one's thinking, feeling, mood, and behavior. Data from the National Institute of Mental Health (NIMH) report that in 2017, there were an estimated 46.6 million adults aged 18 or older in the United States with any mental illness (AMI). This number represented 18.9 percent of all U.S. adults with mental disabilities, which includes conditions in varying degrees of severity.

Mental Disability and Rehabilitation, First Edition focuses on the prevalence, signs and symptoms, diagnosis, and treatment methods of common mental and psychotic disorders. It also discusses co-occurring and affective disorders, including mental-health and substance-use disorders. Information about the personal, social, and economic impact of mental disabilities, mental-health services, recovery, and rehabilitation is included. The legal requirements to qualify for disability status and the rights and benefits of people with mental disabilities are also discussed in detail. The book concludes with a glossary of mental-health terms and a directory of mental-health organizations.

HOW TO USE THIS BOOK

This book is divided into parts and chapters. Parts focus on broad areas of interest. Chapters are devoted to single topics within a part.

Part 1: Psychiatric Disability describes mental disability, tracing early signs and symptoms, and the prevalence of mental illness. It talks about co-occurring disorders and mental health in relation to substance use. It explains how mental health is related to various chronic diseases and elaborates how it affects quality of life (QOL). It also gives insight into different types of mental and psychotic disorders.

Part 2: Personal, Social, and Economic Impact of Mental Disability explains how mental disability affects a person's life, mental health and lifestyle issues, and the link between poverty and mental illness, including social stigma and media portrayal of mental illness. Mental-health interventions at work is also explained in detail.

Part 3: Recovery, Rehabilitation, and Caregiving talks about medical and social approaches to mental-health treatments, such as rehabilitation medicine, psychotherapy, peer support, and integrated care. It gives tips on caring for someone who is mentally disabled and throws light on the future technology to treat mental illness.

Part 4: Protections, Rights, and Benefits talks about legal requirements to qualify for disability status and explains how to access mental-health benefits through the Affordable Care Act (ACA). It highlights the rights of students and employees with mental disabilities, and provides information about the disability rights movement and neurodiversity movement.

Part 5: Additional Resources lists government and private organizations that provide information and services for people with mental disabilities.

BIBLIOGRAPHIC NOTE

This volume contains documents and excerpts from publications issued by the following U.S. government agencies: Administration for Community Living (ACL); Agency for Healthcare Research and Quality (AHRQ); Benefits.gov; Centers for Disease Control and Prevention (CDC); *Eunice Kennedy Shriver* National Institute of Child Health and Human Development (NICHD); National Institute of Mental Health (NIMH); National Institute on Drug Abuse (NIDA); National Institute on Drug Abuse (NIDA) for Teens; National Institutes of Health (NIH); Office of Adolescent Health (OAH), Office of Disease Prevention and Health Promotion (ODPHP); Office of the Assistant Secretary for Planning and Evaluation (ASPE); Office of the Assistant Secretary for Preparedness and Response (ASPR); Office on Women's Health (OWH); Substance Abuse and Mental Health Services Administration (SAMHSA); U.S. Commission on Civil Rights (USCCR); U.S. Department of Education (ED); U.S. Department of Health and Human Services (HHS); U.S. Department of Labor (DOL); U.S. Department of the Interior (DOI); U.S. Department of Veterans Affairs (VA); U.S. Equal Employment Opportunity Commission (EEOC); and U.S. Social Security Administration (SSA).

It may also contain original material produced by Omnigraphics and reviewed by medical consultants.

MEDICAL REVIEW

Omnigraphics contracts with a team of qualified, senior medical professionals who serve as medical consultants for the *Disability Series*. As necessary, medical consultants review reprinted and original written material for currency and accuracy. Citations including the phrase "Reviewed (month, year)" indicate material reviewed by this team. Medical consultation services are provided to the *Disability Series* editors by:

Dr. Vijayalakshmi, MBBS, DGO, MD
Dr. Senthil Selvan, MBBS, DCH, MD
Dr. K. Sivanandham, MBBS, DCH, MS (Research), PhD

ABOUT THE *DISABILITY SERIES*

At the request of librarians serving the one in four Americans who live with a disability and those seeking the information needed to understand, navigate, and manage a disability, the *Disability Series* was developed as a specially focused set of volumes within Omnigraphics' *Health Reference Series*. Each volume deals comprehensively with a topic selected according to the needs and interests of these patrons. The volumes provide the authoritative health information that librarians rely on to arm consumers with the facts they need to take control of their well-being and address and inform themselves about health challenges that they or a family member or loved one are facing. Patrons seeking this information will find answers to their questions in the *Disability Series*. The *Series*, however, is not intended to serve as a tool for diagnosing disability, in prescribing treatments, or as a substitute for the healthcare provider–patient relationship. All people concerned about medical symptoms or the possibility of disability or illness are encouraged to seek professional care from an appropriate healthcare provider.

An accessible *Disability Resource Center* portal will serve as a companion product for this series.

If there is a topic you would like to see addressed in a future volume of the *Disability Series*, please write to:

Managing Editor
Disability Series
Omnigraphics
615 Griswold St., Ste. 520
Detroit, MI 48226

A NOTE ABOUT SPELLING AND STYLE

Disability Series editors use *Stedman's Medical Dictionary* as an authority for questions related to the spelling of medical terms and *The Chicago Manual of Style* for questions related to grammatical structures, punctuation, and other editorial concerns. Consistent adherence is not always possible, however, because the individual volumes within the *Series* include many documents from a wide variety of different producers, and the editor's primary goal is to present material from each source as accurately as possible. This sometimes means that information in different chapters or sections may follow other guidelines and alternate spelling authorities. For example, occasionally a copyright holder may require that eponymous terms be shown in possessive forms (Crohn's disease vs. Crohn disease) or that British spelling norms be retained (leukaemia vs. leukemia).

Part 1 | **Psychiatric Disability**

Chapter 1 | Mental Health and Early Warning Signs

WHAT IS MENTAL HEALTH?

Mental health includes emotional, psychological, and social well-being. It affects how we think, feel, and act. It also helps determine how we handle stress, relate to others, and make choices. Mental health is important at every stage of life, from childhood and adolescence through adulthood.

Over the course of your life, if you experience mental-health problems, your thinking, mood, and behavior could be affected. Many factors contribute to mental-health problems, including:

- Biological factors, such as genes or brain chemistry
- Life experiences, such as trauma or abuse
- Family history of mental-health problems

Mental-health problems are common but help is available. People with mental-health problems can get better and many recover completely.

EARLY WARNING SIGNS

Not sure if you or someone you know is living with mental-health problems? Experiencing one or more of the following feelings or behaviors can be an early warning sign of a problem:

- Eating or sleeping too much or too little
- Pulling away from people and usual activities

This chapter contains text excerpted from the following sources: Text beginning with the heading "What Is Mental Health?" is excerpted from "What Is Mental Health?" MentalHealth.gov, U.S. Department of Health and Human Services (HHS), April 5, 2019; Text beginning with the heading "Why Is Mental Health Important?" is excerpted from "Mental Health and Mental Disorders," Office of Disease Prevention and Health Promotion (ODPHP), U.S. Department of Health and Human Services (HHS), December 7, 2010. Reviewed October 2019.

- Having low or no energy
- Feeling numb or like nothing matters
- Having unexplained aches and pains
- Feeling helpless or hopeless
- Smoking, drinking, or using drugs more than usual
- Feeling unusually confused, forgetful, on edge, angry, upset, worried, or scared
- Yelling or fighting with family and friends
- Experiencing severe mood swings that cause problems in relationships
- Having persistent thoughts and memories you cannot get out of your head
- Hearing voices or believing things that are not true
- Thinking of harming yourself or others
- Inability to perform daily tasks like taking care of your kids or getting to work or school

MENTAL HEALTH AND WELLNESS

Positive mental health allows people to:

- Realize their full potential
- Cope with the stresses of life
- Work productively
- Make meaningful contributions to their communities

Ways to maintain positive mental health include:

- Getting professional help if you need it
- Connecting with others
- Staying positive
- Being physically active
- Helping others
- Getting enough sleep
- Developing coping skills

WHY IS MENTAL HEALTH IMPORTANT?

Mental disorders are among the most common causes of disability. The resulting disease burden of mental illness is among the highest of all diseases. In any given year, an estimated 18.1 percent (43.6

million) of U.S. adults ages 18 years or older suffered from any mental illness and 4.2 percent (9.8 million) suffered from a seriously debilitating mental illness. Neuropsychiatric disorders are the leading cause of disability in the United States, accounting for 18.7 percent of all years of life lost to disability and premature mortality. Moreover, suicide is the tenth leading cause of death in the United States, accounting for the deaths of approximately 43,000 Americans in 2014.

Mental health and physical health are closely connected. Mental health plays a major role in people's ability to maintain good physical health. Mental illnesses, such as depression and anxiety, affect people's ability to participate in health-promoting behaviors. In turn, problems with physical health, such as chronic diseases, can have a serious impact on mental health and decrease a person's ability to participate in treatment and recovery.

UNDERSTANDING MENTAL HEALTH AND MENTAL DISORDERS

The existing model for understanding mental health and mental disorders emphasizes the interaction of social, environmental, and genetic factors throughout the lifespan. In behavioral health, researchers identify:

- Risk factors, which predispose individuals to mental illness
- Protective factors, which protect them from developing mental disorders

Researchers now know that the prevention of mental, emotional, and behavioral (MEB) disorders is inherently interdisciplinary and draws on a variety of different strategies.

Over the past 20 years, research on the prevention of mental disorders has progressed. The understanding of how the brain functions under minimally stressed conditions and in response to stressors, combined with knowledge of how the brain develops over time, has been essential to that progress. The major areas of progress include evidence that:

- MEB disorders are common and begin early in life
- The greatest opportunity for prevention is among young people

- There are multiyear effects of multiple preventive interventions on reducing substance abuse, conduct disorder, antisocial behavior, aggression, and child maltreatment
- The incidence of depression among pregnant women and adolescents can be reduced
- School-based violence prevention can reduce the base rate of aggressive behaviors in an average school by 25 to 33 percent
- There are potential indicated preventive interventions for schizophrenia
- Improving family functioning and positive parenting can have positive outcomes on mental health and can reduce poverty-related risk
- School-based preventive interventions aimed at improving social and emotional outcomes can also improve academic outcomes
- Interventions targeting families dealing with adversities, such as parental depression or divorce, can be effective in reducing the risk for depression among children and increasing effective parenting
- Some preventive interventions have benefits that exceed costs, with the available evidence strongest for early childhood interventions
- Implementation is complex, and it is important that interventions be relevant to the target audiences

The progress identified above has led to a stronger understanding of the importance of protective factors. A 2009 Institute of Medicine (IOM) report advocates for multidisciplinary prevention strategies at the community level that support the development of children in healthy social environments. In addition to advancements in the prevention of mental disorders, there continues to be steady progress in treating mental disorders as new drugs and stronger evidence-based outcomes become available.

EMERGING ISSUES IN MENTAL HEALTH AND MENTAL DISORDERS

New mental-health issues have emerged among some special populations, such as:

- Veterans who have experienced physical and mental trauma
- People in communities with large-scale psychological trauma caused by natural disasters
- Older adults, as the understanding and treatment of dementia and mood disorders continues to improve

As the federal government begins to implement the health-reform legislation, it will give attention to providing services for individuals with mental illness and substance-use disorders (SUDs), including new opportunities for access to and coverage for treatment and prevention services.

Chapter 2 | Mental Disorders

WHAT ARE MENTAL DISORDERS?

Mental disorders (or mental illnesses) are conditions that affect your thinking, feeling, mood, and behavior. They may be occasional or long-lasting (chronic). They can affect your ability to relate to others and function each day.

WHAT ARE SOME TYPES OF MENTAL DISORDERS?

There are many different types of mental disorders. Some common ones include:

- Anxiety disorders, including panic disorder, obsessive-compulsive disorder (OCD), posttraumatic stress disorder (PTSD), and phobias
- Depression, bipolar disorder, and other mood disorders
- Eating disorders
- Personality disorders
- Psychotic disorders, including schizophrenia

WHAT CAUSES MENTAL DISORDERS

There is no single cause for mental illness. A number of factors can contribute to risk for mental illness, such as:

- Your genes and family history
- Your life experiences, such as stress or a history of abuse, especially if they happen in childhood
- Biological factors such as chemical imbalances in the brain
- A traumatic brain injury
- A mother's exposure to viruses or toxic chemicals while pregnant
- Use of alcohol or recreational drugs

This chapter includes text excerpted from "Mental Disorders," MedlinePlus, National Institutes of Health (NIH), September 15,2014. Reviewed October 2019.

- Having a serious medical condition like cancer
- Having few friends, and feeling lonely or isolated

Mental disorders are not caused by character flaws. They have nothing to do with being lazy or weak.

WHO IS AT RISK FOR MENTAL DISORDERS?

Mental disorders are common. More than half of all Americans will be diagnosed with a mental disorder at some time in their life.

HOW ARE MENTAL DISORDERS DIAGNOSED?

The steps to getting a diagnosis include the following:

- A medical history
- A physical exam and possibly lab tests, if your provider thinks that other medical conditions could be causing your symptoms
- A psychological evaluation. You will answer questions about your thinking, feelings, and behaviors.

WHAT ARE THE TREATMENTS FOR MENTAL DISORDERS?

Treatment depends on which mental disorder you have and how serious it is. You and your provider will work on a treatment plan just for you. It usually involves some type of therapy. You may also take medicines. Some people also need social support and education on managing their condition.

In some cases, you may need more intensive treatment. You may need to go to a psychiatric hospital. This could be because your mental illness is severe. Or it could be because you are at risk of hurting yourself or someone else. In the hospital, you will get counseling, group discussions, and activities with mental-health professionals and other patients.

Chapter 3 | Prevalence of Mental Illness

MENTAL ILLNESS: AN OVERVIEW

Mental illnesses are common in the United States. Nearly one in five U.S. adults live with a mental illness (46.6 million in 2017). Mental illnesses include many different conditions that vary in degree of severity, ranging from mild to moderate to severe. Two broad categories can be used to describe these conditions: any mental illness (AMI) and serious mental illness (SMI). AMI encompasses all recognized mental illnesses. SMI is a smaller and more severe subset of AMI.

Any Mental Illness

Any mental illness is defined as "a mental, behavioral, or emotional disorder." AMI can vary in impact, ranging from no impairment to mild, moderate, and even severe impairment (e.g., individuals with serious mental illness as defined below).

Serious Mental Illness

Serious mental illness is defined as "a mental, behavioral, or emotional disorder resulting in serious functional impairment, which substantially interferes with or limits one or more major life activities." The burden of mental illnesses is particularly concentrated among those who experience disability due to SMI.

PREVALENCE OF ANY MENTAL DISORDER AMONG ADULTS

How Common Is Any Mental Illness?

Figure 3.1 shows the past-year prevalence of AMI among U.S. adults.

This chapter includes text excerpted from "Mental Illness," National Institute of Mental Health (NIMH), February 2019.

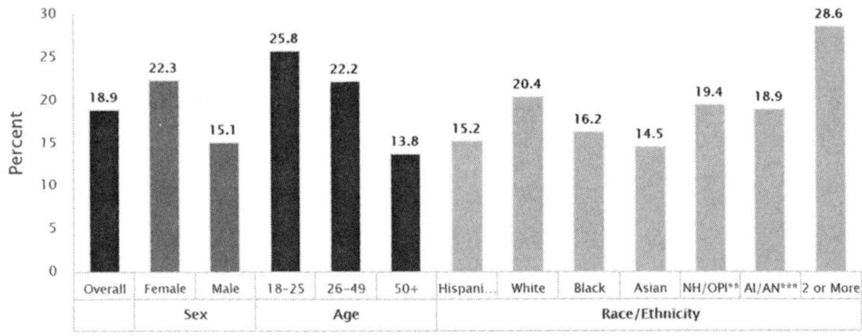

Figure 3.1. Past Year Prevalence of Any Mental Illness among U.S. Adults (2017). *(Source: Substance Abuse and Mental Health Services Administration (SAMHSA).)*

*All other groups are non-Hispanic or Latinx. **NH/OPI = Native Hawaiian/Other Pacific Islander. ***AI/AN = American Indian/Alaskan Native

- In 2017, there were an estimated 46.6 million adults aged 18 or older in the United States with AMI. This number represented 18.9 percent of all U.S. adults.
- The prevalence of AMI was higher among women (22.3%) than men (15.1%).
- Young adults aged 18 to 25 years had the highest prevalence of AMI (25.8%) compared to adults aged 26 to 49 years (22.2%) and aged 50 and older (13.8%).
- The prevalence of AMI was highest among adults reporting two or more races (28.6%), followed by White adults (20.4%). The prevalence of AMI was lowest among Asian adults (14.5%).

Mental-Health Services: Any Mental Illness

Figure 3.2 presents data on mental-health services received within the past year by U.S. adults aged 18 or older with any AMI. The National Survey on Drug Use and Health (NSDUH) defines mental-health services as "having received inpatient treatment/counseling or outpatient treatment/counseling or having used prescription medication for problems with emotions, nerves, or mental health."

- In 2017, among the 46.6 million adults with AMI, 19.8 million (42.6%) received mental-health services in the past year.

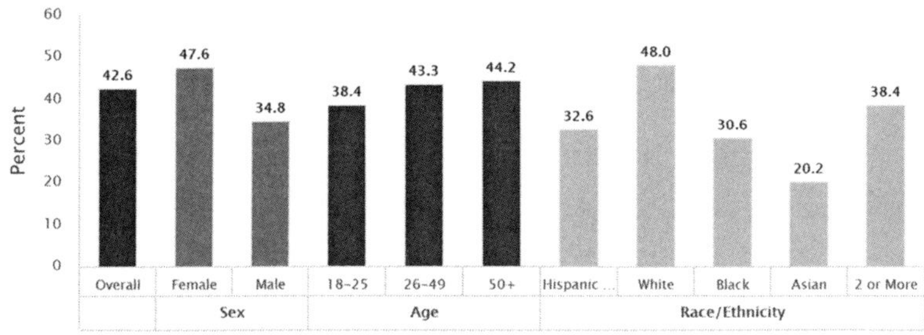

Figure 3.2. Mental-Health Services Received in Past Year among U.S. Adults with Any Mental Illness (2017). *(Source: Substance Abuse and Mental Health Services Administration (SAMHSA).)*

*All other groups are non-Hispanic or Latinx.

- More women with AMI (47.6%) received mental-health services than men with AMI (34.8%).
- The percentage of young adults aged 18 to 25 years with AMI who received mental-health services (38.4%) was lower than adults with AMI aged 26 to 49 years (43.3%) and aged 50 and older (44.2%).

How Common Is Serious Mental Illness?

Figure 3.3 shows the past year prevalence of SMI among U.S. adults.

- In 2017, there were an estimated 11.2 million adults aged 18 or older in the United States with SMI. This number represented 4.5 percent of all U.S. adults.
- The prevalence of SMI was higher among women (5.7%) than men (3.3%).
- Young adults aged 18 to 25 years had the highest prevalence of SMI (7.5%) compared to adults aged 26 to 49 years (5.6%) and aged 50 and older (2.7%).
- The prevalence of SMI was highest among the adults reporting two or more races (8.1%), followed by White adults (5.2%). The prevalence of SMI was lowest among Asian adults (2.4%).

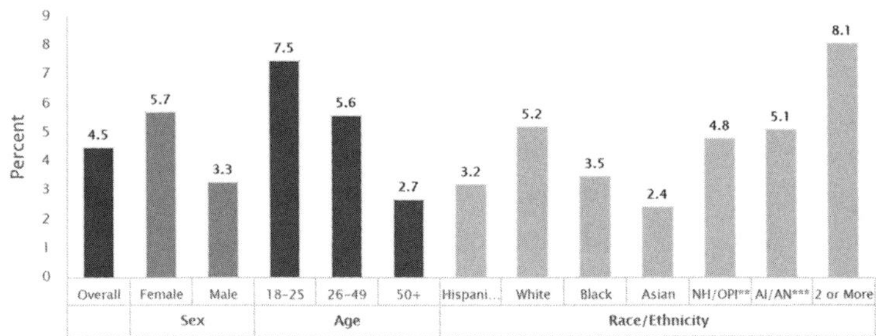

Figure 3.3. Past Year Prevalence of Serious Mental Illness among U.S. Adults (2017). *(Source: Substance Abuse and Mental Health Services Administration (SAMHSA).)*

*All other groups are non-Hispanic or Latinx. **NH/OPI = Native Hawaiian/Other Pacific Islander. ***AI/AN = American Indian/Alaskan Native

Mental-Health Services: Serious Mental Illness

Figure 3.4 presents data on mental-health services received within the past year by U.S. adults 18 or older with SMIs. The NSDUH defines mental-health services as having received inpatient treatment/counseling or outpatient treatment/counseling or having used prescription medication for problems with emotions, nerves, or mental health.

- In 2017, among the 11.2 million adults with SMI, 7.5 million (66.7%) received mental-health treatment in the past year.
- More women with SMI (71.5%) received mental-health treatment than men with SMI (57.7%).
- The percentage of young adults aged 18 to 25 years with SMI who received mental-health treatment (57.4%) was lower than adults with SMI aged 26 to 49 years (66.2%) and aged 50 and older (75.6%).

PREVALENCE OF ANY MENTAL DISORDER AMONG ADOLESCENTS

Based on diagnostic interview data from the National Comorbidity Survey Adolescent Supplement (NCS-A), Figure 3.5 shows the lifetime prevalence of any mental disorder among U.S. adolescents aged 13 to 18.

- An estimated 49.5 percent of adolescents had any mental disorder.

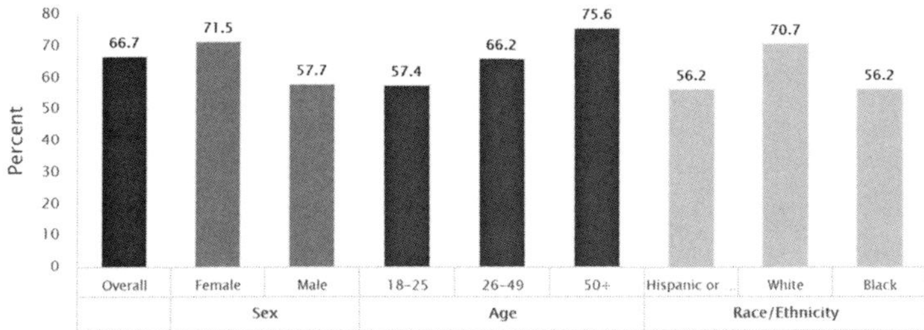

Figure 3.4. Mental-Health Services Received in Past Year among U.S. Adults with Serious Mental Illness (2017). *(Source: Substance Abuse and Mental Health Services Administration (SAMHSA).)*

*All other groups are non-Hispanic or Latinx.

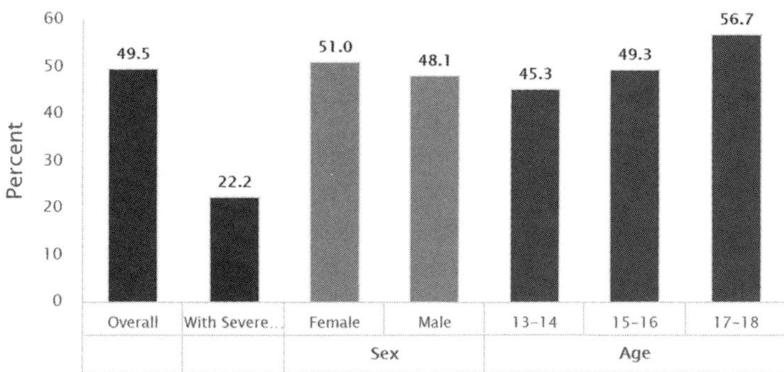

Figure 3.5. Lifetime Prevalence of Any Mental Disorder among Adolescents (2001–2004). *(Source: National Comorbidity Survey Adolescent Supplement (NCS-A).)*

- Of adolescents with any mental disorder, an estimated 22.2 percent had severe impairment. *Diagnostic and Statistical Manual of Mental Disorders* (*DSM-IV*) based criteria were used to determine impairment level.

Chapter 4 | What Are Co-Occurring Disorders?

CO-OCCURRING DISORDERS

When a person has mental-health and substance use disorder at the same time, they have co-occurring disorders. Compared to the general population, people with mental-health disorders are more likely to experience a substance-use disorder, repeatedly use alcohol and/or drugs to the point of impairment, and neglect major responsibilities at home, work, or school. Youth who have experienced a major depressive episode are twice as likely to start using alcohol or an illicit drug. A 2010 study found that more than 29 percent of youth who started using alcohol within the past year did so after a major depressive episode, compared to 14.5 percent of youth who had not experienced a major depressive episode. The same pattern also occurred with the use of illicit drugs.

Substance use shares many characteristics with mental illness. Prevention efforts and early treatment are beneficial for people who are at risk for both substance-use and mental-health disorders. A U.S. Surgeon General's report highlights the scope of substance use (including alcohol) and its negative health impacts for individuals and the nation. Because mental-health and substance-use disorders are complicated and involve biological, psychological, and social elements, the Substance Abuse and Mental Health Services Administration (SAMHSA) supports an integrated treatment approach to co-occurring disorders. This approach allows practitioners to

This chapter contains text excerpted from the following sources: Text under the heading "Co-Occurring Disorders" is excerpted from "Common Mental Health Disorders in Adolescence," U.S. Department of Health and Human Services (HHS), May 1, 2019; Text beginning with the heading "Which Came First?" is excerpted from "What Are "Co-Occurring" Disorders?" National Institute on Drug Abuse (NIDA) for Teens, March 8, 2012. Reviewed October 2019.

comprehensively address symptoms and underlying causes, which often lowers the cost of treatment and leads to better outcomes.

Substance use is not the only disorder that occurs at the same time as mental-health disorders. Different mental-health disorders can occur together (such as anxiety and depression) or mental-health disorders can overlap with physical health disorders (such as depression and diabetes). Symptoms of mental-health disorders can also be similar to other conditions. For example, autism spectrum disorder (ASD) is the name for a group of developmental disorders often characterized by impairments in the ability to communicate and interact with others. ASD includes a wide range of symptoms, skills, and levels of disability. These disorders occur in about 1.5 percent of children and often co-occur with disorders such as depression, anxiety, and sensory integration disorder.

WHICH CAME FIRST

It is often impossible to say which disorder came first. In one case, a person may experience anxiety from childhood trauma and turn to drugs to cope, developing an addiction. In another case, the person may use heroin and have negative experiences that could lead to posttraumatic stress disorder (PTSD). The important thing is to get help for both problems—substance-use problems and any other mental-health disorders.

Treating co-occurring disorders can be challenging because often the different specialists involved do not coordinate treatment for the different problems. Doctors, social workers, psychologists, and psychiatrists most often treat mental-health disorders, whereas a mix of healthcare professionals with various backgrounds may provide treatment for drug addiction.

TREATMENT MUST ADDRESS THE WHOLE PERSON

National Institute on Drug Abuse (NIDA) and other federal agencies are working to make sure people who have co-occurring disorders receive integrated treatment that addresses both substance use and other mental-health disorders. Some medications may ease symptoms of a mental-health disorder and also may help the person stay off a certain drug.

Other types of treatment also may be effective. For example, for teens with co-occurring disorders, cognitive-behavioral therapy (CBT) can help. This therapy helps the person change harmful beliefs and behaviors, and provides skills to handle stressful circumstances.

Chapter 5 | The Connection between Mental Health and Chronic Disease

CHRONIC DISEASES

Chronic diseases are noncommunicable illnesses that are prolonged in duration, do not resolve spontaneously, and are rarely cured completely. They are the leading cause of death and disability in the United States. They cause 7 out of 10 deaths each year and are among the most preventable and treatable of all health problems. Chronic diseases include illnesses such as heart disease, diabetes, cancer, and arthritis.

Mental-health disorders are medical conditions that disrupt a person's thinking, feeling, mood, ability to relate to others, and daily functioning. They are medical conditions that often result in a reduced ability to cope with the routine daily activities such as going to work or raising a family. Just like chronic diseases, mental-health disorders are treatable. Most people diagnosed with a serious mental-health disorder can receive relief from their symptoms by following a treatment plan specifically designed for them by a trained psychologist or psychiatrist. Mental-health disorders are not exclusive to those who exhibit a lack of personal strength, personality traits such as being shy, or have a certain socioeconomic status. Mental-health disorders include illnesses, such as major depression,

This chapter contains text excerpted from the following sources: Text beginning with the heading "Chronic Diseases" is excerpted from "Mental Health and Chronic Diseases," Centers for Disease Control and Prevention (CDC), October 2012. Reviewed October 2019; Text beginning with the heading "Chronic Medical Conditions and the Risk of Depression" is excerpted from "Chronic Illness and Mental Health: Recognizing and Treating Depression," National Institute of Mental Health (NIMH), December 18, 2015. Reviewed October 2019.

bipolar disorder, obsessive-compulsive disorder (OCD), and post-traumatic stress disorder (PTSD).

One common finding is that people who suffer from chronic disease are more likely to also suffer from depression. Scientists have yet to determine if having a chronic disease increases the prevalence of depression or depression increases the risk of obtaining a chronic disease. Regardless of the cause, chronic diseases and mental-health disorders are treatable and employers can use multiple strategies to make their work environments more supportive of overall physical and mental health and general well-being.

RELATIONSHIP BETWEEN MENTAL HEALTH, CHRONIC DISEASE, AND INJURY

Both mental-health disorders and chronic diseases are common and disabling. These conditions can affect anyone, regardless of age, culture, race/ethnicity, gender, or income. In 2009, 145 million people—almost half of all Americans—were living with a chronic condition. Approximately 26 percent of American adults aged 18 years and older suffer from a diagnosable mental disorder in a given year. Arthritis, as a chronic condition, and depression, as a mental-health illness, are both leading causes of disability worldwide.

Many other associations exist between mental illness and cardiovascular disease, diabetes, obesity, asthma, and arthritis, to name a few. Major depressive disorder (MDD) and other common chronic diseases are prevalent. Depression is found to co-occur in 17 percent of cardiovascular cases, 23 percent of cerebrovascular cases, 27 percent of diabetes patients, and more than 40 percent of individuals with cancer. The relationship between mental health, chronic disease, and injury is significant. Many examples exist of individuals with a chronic condition or risk factor and an increased risk for mental illness such as the risk for tobacco use is about twice as high for those with mental illness compared to the general population. Injuries both intentional, such as homicide and suicide, and unintentional, such as motor vehicle accidents, are 2 to 6 times higher for persons with a history of mental illness than those without a history.

Table 5.1. Mental Health and Chronic Diseases

Mental Health	**Chronic Disease**	
Risk Factors	**Modifiable Risk Factors**	**Nonmodifiable Risk Factors**
Family history	Poor eating habits	Age
Stressful life conditions	Lack of physical activity	Family history
Having a chronic disease	Tobacco use	
Traumatic experience	Excessive alcohol use	
Use of illegal drugs	Environmental factors	
Childhood abuse or neglect	Socioeconomic status	
Lack of social support		

WHAT CAUSES MENTAL-HEALTH DISORDERS AND CHRONIC DISEASES

While the causes of mental-health disorders are unknown, there are certain factors that can increase an individual's risk of developing a mental-health disorder. The risks and causes of chronic diseases are much more well-established. Below is a list of the common risk factors for mental health and chronic diseases:

CHRONIC MEDICAL CONDITIONS AND THE RISK OF DEPRESSION

The same factors that increase risk of depression in otherwise healthy people also raise the risk in people with other medical illnesses. These risk factors include a personal or family history of depression or loss of family members to suicide.

However, there are some risk factors directly related to having another illness. For example, conditions such as Parkinson disease and stroke cause changes in the brain. In some cases, these changes may have a direct role in depression. Illness-related anxiety and stress can also trigger symptoms of depression.

PEOPLE WITH DEPRESSION ARE AT HIGHER RISK FOR OTHER MEDICAL CONDITIONS

It may have come as no surprise that people with a medical illness or condition are more likely to suffer from depression. The reverse is also true: the risk of developing some physical illnesses is higher in people with depression.

People with depression have an increased risk of cardiovascular disease, diabetes, stroke, and Alzheimer disease, for example. Research also suggests that people with depression are at higher risk for osteoporosis relative to others. The reasons are not yet clear. One factor with some of these illnesses is that many people with depression may have less access to good medical care. They may have a harder time caring for their health, for example, seeking care, taking prescribed medication, eating well, and exercising.

Ongoing research is also exploring whether physiological changes seen in depression may play a role in increasing the risk of physical illness. In people with depression, scientists have found changes in the way several different systems in the body function, all of which can have an impact on physical health:

- Signs of increased inflammation
- Changes in the control of heart rate and blood circulation
- Abnormalities in stress hormones
- Metabolic changes typical of those seen in people at risk for diabetes

Chapter 6 | The Connection between Mental Illness and Substance-Use Disorders

DRUGS AND ALCOHOL

Did you know that addiction to drugs or alcohol is a mental illness? Substance-use disorder (SUD) changes normal desires and priorities. It changes normal behaviors and interferes with the ability to work, go to school, and to have good relationships with friends and family. In 2014, 20.2 million adults in the United States had an SUD and 7.9 million had both an SUD and another mental illness. More than half of the people with both an SUD and another mental illness were men (4.1 million). Having two illnesses at the same time is known as "comorbidity" and it can make treating each disorder more difficult.

TOBACCO

Tobacco is another substance associated with addiction and health risks. Tobacco can be smoked, chewed or sniffed. However, the most common way people consume tobacco is by smoking cigarettes. Research has shown that adults with mental illness are more likely to smoke cigarettes than other adults. This is particularly true among people with major depression and those diagnosed with

This chapter contains text excerpted from the following sources: Text beginning with the heading "Drugs and Alcohol" is excerpted from "Substance Use and Mental Health," National Institute of Mental Health (NIMH), May 2016. Reviewed October 2019; Text beginning with the heading "Drug Use and Mental-Health Disorders in Childhood or Adolescence Increases Later Risk" is excerpted from "The Connection between Substance Use Disorders and Mental Illness," National Institute on Drug Abuse (NIDA), February 2018; Text under the heading "Diagnosing Mental Health and Substance-Use Disorder" is excerpted from "Mental Health and Substance Use Disorders," Substance Abuse and Mental Health Services Administration (SAMHSA), April 13, 2019.

schizophrenia. It is estimated that people with psychiatric disorders purchase approximately 44 percent of all cigarettes sold in the United States. Smoking is believed to be one reason that individuals with mental illnesses have more physical health problems and die younger than people without a mental illness.

DRUG USE AND MENTAL-HEALTH DISORDERS IN CHILDHOOD OR ADOLESCENCE INCREASES LATER RISK

The brain continues to develop through adolescence. Circuits that control executive functions such as decision-making and impulse control are among the last to mature, a reality which enhances vulnerability to drug use and the development of a SUD. Early drug use is a strong risk factor for later development of SUDs, and it may also be a risk factor for the later occurrence of other mental illnesses. However, this link is not necessarily causative and may reflect shared risk factors including genetic vulnerability, psychosocial experiences, and/or general environmental influences. For example, frequent marijuana use during adolescence can increase the risk of psychosis in adulthood, specifically in individuals who carry a particular gene variant.

It is also true that having a mental disorder in childhood or adolescence can increase the risk of later drug use and the development of a SUD. Some research has found that mental illness may precede a SUD, suggesting that a better diagnosis of youth mental illness may help reduce comorbidity. One study found that adolescent-onset bipolar disorder confers a greater risk of subsequent SUD compared to adult-onset bipolar disorder. Similarly, other research suggests that youth develop internalizing disorders, including depression and anxiety, prior to developing SUDs.

UNTREATED CHILDHOOD ATTENTION DEFICIT HYPERACTIVITY DISORDER CAN INCREASE LATER RISK OF DRUG PROBLEMS

Numerous studies have documented an increased risk for SUDs in youth with untreated ADHD, although some studies suggest that only those with comorbid conduct disorders have greater odds of later developing an SUD. Given this linkage, it is important to determine whether effective treatment of ADHD could prevent subsequent drug use and addiction. Treatment of childhood ADHD with stimulant medications such as methylphenidate or amphetamine reduces impulsive behavior, fidgeting, and the inability to concentrate that characterize ADHD.

That risk presents a challenge when treating children with ADHD, since effective treatment often involves prescribing stimulant medications with addictive potential. Although the research is not yet conclusive, many studies suggest that ADHD medications do not increase the risk of SUD among children with this condition. It is important to combine stimulant medication for ADHD with appropriate family and child education and behavioral interventions, including counseling on the chronic nature of ADHD and risk for SUD.

DIAGNOSING MENTAL-HEALTH AND SUBSTANCE-USE DISORDER

The Substance Abuse and Mental Health Services Administration works to reduce the impact of the most common mental health and SUDs on America's communities.

Mental health and SUDs affect people from all walks of life and all age groups. These illnesses are common, recurrent, and often serious, but they are treatable and many people do recover. Mental disorders involve changes in thinking, mood, and/or behavior. These disorders can affect how we relate to others and make choices. Reaching a level that can be formally diagnosed often depends on a reduction in a person's ability to function as a result of the disorder. For example:

- Serious mental illness (SMI) is defined as someone over 18, having (within the past year) a diagnosable mental, behavior, or emotional disorder that causes serious functional impairment that substantially interferes with or limits one or more major life activities.
- For people under the age of 18, the term "serious emotional disturbance" refers to a diagnosable mental, behavioral, or emotional disorder in the past year, which resulted in functional impairment that substantially interferes with or limits the child's role or functioning in the family, school, or community activities.

- Substance-use disorders occur when the recurrent use of alcohol and/or drugs causes clinically significant impairment, including health problems, disability, and failure to meet major responsibilities at work, school, or home.

Chapter 7 | **Mental Illness and Life Expectancy**

COMBATING EARLY DEATH IN PEOPLE WITH SERIOUS MENTAL ILLNESS

An article and commentary in the *Journal of the American Medical Association Psychiatry* contain some disturbing statistics about early death for people with a serious mental illness (SMI). Mark Olfson's team followed a group of 1.1 million people with schizophrenia and found that, during the study period, they were more than 3.5 times more likely to die than the general population. These individuals are estimated to be losing 28.5 years of life, primarily because of natural causes. Eighty-five percent of the premature deaths were due to largely preventable conditions, such as high blood pressure, high cholesterol, diabetes, and heart disease.

Premature death among people with SMI, including schizophrenia, has been recognized for some time. It is also known that unhealthy lifestyle behaviors such as poor diet, lack of exercise, and smoking contribute to many of their physical problems. People with schizophrenia are much more likely to smoke than people with no mental illness.

The Olfson et al. paper and the accompanying commentary identify the need to concentrate on risk factors related to unhealthy lifestyle, the need to treat these health risk factors, and the need to manage physical illnesses that are common in people with schizophrenia such as diabetes and heart disease.

This chapter includes text excerpted from "Combating Early Death in People with Serious Mental Illness," National Institute of Mental Health (NIMH), November 4, 2015. Reviewed October 2019.

WHAT IS THE NATIONAL INSTITUTE OF MENTAL HEALTH DOING ABOUT THIS ISSUE?

Several years ago, the National Institute of Mental Health (NIMH) launched a large research initiative on ways to prevent and treat these health problems in people with schizophrenia and other SMIs. Currently, the institute funds more than a dozen studies to accomplish that goal. These studies focus mainly on cardiometabolic problems, problems that affect the heart and blood and contribute to early mortality.

Dr. Susan Azrin, program chief of the Primary Care Research Program in NIMH's Division of Services and Intervention Research, says, "The premature death of people with SMI, due mainly to preventable causes, is a tremendous public health concern. Effective strategies to reduce common health risk factors, such as high blood pressure, poor diet, and fitness, and smoking, are available to the general population. We need to figure out how to make these effective strategies available to people with SMIs at the earliest opportunity."

The National Institute of Mental Health's (NIMH) research effort aims to reach people with SMI earlier in life before these dangerous health problems take hold. In 2016, NIMH supported five new research projects that developed and tested new approaches for reducing cardiometabolic risks in youth with serious emotional disturbance and young adults with serious mental illness.

Chapter 8 | Psychiatric Disability and Quality of Life

"Quality of life" is often described as the degree of satisfaction one feels with one's overall station in life and her or his sense of well-being. Studies indicate that people with a mental disability are more likely to suffer from a reduced quality of life (QOL) than members of the overall population. Historically, less attention has been paid to treating the long-term outcomes of chronic illness. This trend is gradually changing, however, and today's comprehensive health-treatment plans include an examination of and strategic effort to improve the overall quality of life of people living with a mental disability, for which a cure has yet to be found.

THE EFFECTS OF PSYCHIATRIC DISABILITY ON QUALITY OF LIFE

The quality of life of a person with a psychiatric disability is determined by reviewing one's individual characteristics, overall life situations, and level of socioeconomic stability. A person with a psychiatric disability, especially one with a diagnosis of schizophrenia, is more likely to experience social isolation, strained interpersonal relationships, unemployment, meager financial means, and an inability to perform many activities associated with everyday living. Symptoms of the illness and its overall side effects can further reduce QOL. Specific areas in which a psychiatric disability can affect QOL are outlined below.

Distress from Symptoms

Distress associated with psychological disability can be defined as "burdensome, painful, and tormenting thoughts and experiences that can overwhelm a person and negatively impact their life." Symptoms such as these interfere with one's everyday life and make it difficult to accomplish daily activities. People in psychological distress mostly concentrate on coping with rather than enjoying their lives.

Experience of Psychosis or Mania

Symptoms, such as hallucinations, delusions, disorientation, and feelings of discomfort, irritability, and agitation are widely observed among people with a psychiatric disability. These symptoms can hinder psychological stability by affecting the behavior, concentration, memory, and decision-making abilities of a person experiencing psychosis or mania, which negatively impact their QOL.

Depressed Mood

Depression is associated with many types of mental illnesses, and acute depression can cause a person to feel not only the sadness and unhappiness associated with depression, but to feel hopeless and suicidal. People diagnosed with a bipolar disorder, in particular, tend to experience heightened levels of distress and depression.

These factors also negatively impact QOL.

Fear and Anxiety

Fear and anxiety are also experienced by many people with a psychiatric disability, and most commonly present in people being treated for schizophrenia, and bipolar or panic disorder. Studies indicate that, even when a patient is able to reach a state of equilibrium, they live in fear of relapse, especially when financial worries restrict their ability to plan for the future.

Energy and Motivation

Research suggests that depression can produce a lack of energy and motivation in individuals affected by it. Although energy and motivation are two different experiences (one physical and the other psychological, respectively) they are closely related. Studies indicate that, in populations that report diminished energy and sense of motivation, these symptoms are primarily the result of the side effects of the medication used to treat their psychological illness.

Well-Being

Studies further indicate that people with a psychological disability are more likely to report an overall increased sense of satisfaction, well-being, calmness, safety, and feeling of health when they receive ongoing treatment for their disability.

CONTROL, INDEPENDENCE, AND CHOICE

Studies indicate that, as with any member of the population, a person with a psychiatric disability considers it important to have control over her or his overall QOL, and improving this QOL is of immense important to them.

Some external resources that can enhance an overall feeling of control and choice include medication, knowledge, ongoing health-care services, and a sense of financial stability. Personal health, self-confidence, and self-sufficiency are also important elements that can contribute to a positive QOL.

Important things that help a person experience QOL include:

- Positive relationships with friends, family, and a partner
- A secure and consistent living situation
- Daily plans in place that allow one to look forward to living her or his life
- Staying healthy
- Financial security

Improving a patient's quality of life is a primary goal of quality psychiatric care, particularly because many symptoms of psychiatric disabilities are difficult to cure. Hence, a focus on improving an individual's overall quality of life is vital.

References

1. "Quality of Life," Foundation for People with Learning Disabilities (FPLD), August 30, 2015.
2. "Quality of Life of People with Mental Health Problems: A Synthesis of Qualitative Research," BioMed Central Ltd (BMC), November 22, 2012.
3. "Quality of Life in Psychiatric Disorders," Open Access (OA) Text, December 17, 2018.

Chapter 9 | **Common Mental Disorders**

ANXIETY DISORDERS

Fear and anxiety are part of life. You may feel anxious before you take a test or walk down a dark street. This kind of anxiety is useful—it can make you more alert or careful. It usually ends soon after you are out of the situation that caused it. But, for millions of people in the United States, the anxiety does not go away, and gets worse over time.

This chapter contains text excerpted from the following sources: Text under the heading "Anxiety Disorders" is excerpted from "Anxiety," MedlinePlus, National Institutes of Health (NIH), November 4, 2016. Reviewed October 2019; Text under the heading "Attention Deficit Hyperactivity Disorder" is excerpted from "What Is ADHD?" Centers for Disease Control and Prevention (CDC), August 26, 2019; Text under the heading "Autism Spectrum Disorder" is excerpted from "What Is Autism Spectrum Disorder?" Centers for Disease Control and Prevention (CDC), August 27, 2019; Text under the heading "Bipolar Disorder in Children and Teens" is excerpted from "Bipolar Disorder in Children and Teens," National Institute of Mental Health (NIMH), 2015. Reviewed October 2019; Text under the heading "Bipolar Disorder in Adults" is excerpted from "Bipolar Disorder," National Institute of Mental Health (NIMH), November 2017; Text under the heading "Borderline Personality Disorder" is excerpted from "Borderline Personality Disorder," National Institute of Mental Health (NIMH), December 2017; Text under the heading "Depression" is excerpted from "Depression," MedlinePlus, National Institutes of Health (NIH), November 4, 2016. Reviewed October 2019; Text under the heading "Disruptive Behavior Disorders" is excerpted from "Treating Disruptive Behavior Disorders in Children and Teens," Effective Health Care Program, Agency for Healthcare Research and Quality (AHRQ), August 31, 2016. Reviewed October 2019; Text under the heading "Disruptive Mood Dysregulation Disorder" is excerpted from "Disruptive Mood Dysregulation Disorder," National Institute of Mental Health (NIMH), January 2017; Text under the heading "Eating Disorders" is excerpted from "Eating Disorders," MedlinePlus, National Institutes of Health (NIH), March 11, 2016. Reviewed October 2019; Text under the heading "Generalized Anxiety Disorder" is excerpted from "Generalized Anxiety Disorder: When Worry Gets out of Control," National Institute of Mental Health (NIMH), 2016. Reviewed October 2019; Text under the heading "Obsessive-Compulsive Disorder" is excerpted from "Obsessive-Compulsive Disorder: When Unwanted Thoughts or Irresistible Actions Take Over," MedlinePlus, National Institute of Mental Health (NIMH), 2016. Reviewed October 2019; Text under the heading "Personality Disorders" is excerpted from "Personality Disorders," MedlinePlus, National Institutes of Health (NIH), December 2, 2016. Reviewed October 2019; Text under the heading "Posttraumatic Stress Disorders" is excerpted from "Posttraumatic Stress Disorders," MedlinePlus, National Institutes of Health (NIH), August 11, 2016. Reviewed October 2019.

They may have chest pains or nightmares. They may even be afraid to leave home. These people have anxiety disorders. Types include:

- Panic disorder
- Obsessive-compulsive disorder (OCD)
- Posttraumatic stress disorder (PTSD
- Phobias
- Generalized anxiety disorder (GAD)

Treatment can involve medicines, therapy, or both.

ATTENTION DEFICIT HYPERACTIVITY DISORDER

Attention deficit hyperactivity disorder (ADHD) is one of the most common neurodevelopmental disorders of childhood. It is usually first diagnosed in childhood and often lasts into adulthood. Children with ADHD may have trouble paying attention, controlling impulsive behaviors (may act without thinking about what the result will be), or be overly active.

In most cases, ADHD is best treated with a combination of behavior therapy and medication. For preschool-aged children (four to five years of age) with ADHD, behavior therapy, particularly training for parents, is recommended as the first line of treatment before medication is tried. What works best can depend on the child and family. Good treatment plans will include close monitoring, follow-ups, and making changes, if needed, along the way.

AUTISM SPECTRUM DISORDER

Autism spectrum disorder (ASD) is a developmental disability that can cause significant social, communication, and behavioral challenges. There is often nothing about how people with ASD look that sets them apart from other people, but people with ASD may communicate, interact, behave, and learn in ways that are different from most other people. The learning, thinking, and problem-solving abilities of people with ASD can range from gifted to severely challenged. Some people with ASD need a lot of help in their daily lives; others need less.

There is currently no cure for ASD. However, research shows that early intervention treatment services can improve a child's development. Early intervention services help children from birth to 3 years old (36 months) learn important skills. Services can include therapy to help the child talk, walk, and interact with others. Therefore, it is important to talk to your child's doctor as soon as possible if you think your child has ASD or other developmental disorder.

BIPOLAR DISORDER IN CHILDREN AND TEENS

Bipolar disorder is a serious brain illness. It is also called "manic-depressive illness" or "manic depression." Children with bipolar disorder go through unusual mood changes. Sometimes they feel very happy or "up," and are much more energetic and active than usual, or than other kids their age. This is called a "manic episode." Sometimes children with bipolar disorder feel very sad and "down," and are much less active than usual. This is called "depression" or a "depressive episode."

Bipolar disorder is not the same as the normal ups and downs every kid goes through. Bipolar symptoms are more powerful than that. The mood swings are more extreme and are accompanied by changes in sleep, energy level, and the ability to think clearly. Bipolar symptoms are so strong that they can make it hard for a child to do well in school or get along with friends and family members. The disorder can also be dangerous. Some young people with bipolar disorder try to hurt themselves or attempt suicide.

Children and teens with bipolar disorder should get treatment. With help, they can manage their symptoms and lead successful lives.

BIPOLAR DISORDER IN ADULTS

Bipolar disorder, sometimes referred to as manic-depressive disorder, is characterized by dramatic shifts in mood, energy, and activity levels that affect a person's ability to carry out day-to-day tasks. These shifts in mood and energy levels are more severe than the normal ups and downs that are experienced by everyone.

BORDERLINE PERSONALITY DISORDER

Borderline personality disorder is an illness marked by an ongoing pattern of varying moods, self-image, and behavior. These symptoms often result in impulsive actions and problems in relationships. People with borderline personality disorder may experience intense episodes of anger, depression, and anxiety that can last from a few hours to days.

Borderline personality disorder has historically been viewed as difficult to treat. But, with newer, evidence-based treatment, many people with the disorder experience fewer or less severe symptoms, and an improved quality of life. It is important that people with borderline personality disorder receive evidence-based, specialized treatment from an appropriately trained provider. Other types of treatment, or treatment provided by a doctor or therapist who is not appropriately trained, may not benefit the person.

DEPRESSION

Depression is a serious medical illness. It is more than just a feeling of being sad or "blue" for a few days. If you are one of the more than 19 million teens and adults in the United States who have depression, the feelings do not go away. They persist and interfere with your everyday life. Symptoms can include:

- Feeling sad or "empty"
- Loss of interest in favorite activities
- Overeating, or not wanting to eat at all
- Not being able to sleep, or sleeping too much
- Feeling very tired
- Feeling hopeless, irritable, anxious, or guilty
- Aches or pains, headaches, cramps, or digestive problems
- Thoughts of death or suicide

Depression is a disorder of the brain. There are a variety of causes, including genetic, biological, environmental, and psychological factors. Depression can happen at any age, but it often begins in teens and young adults. It is much more common in women. Women can also get postpartum depression after the birth of a baby. Some people get seasonal affective disorder in the winter. Depression is one part of bipolar disorder.

There are effective treatments for depression, including antidepressants, talk therapy, or both.

DISRUPTIVE BEHAVIORAL DISORDERS

Disruptive behavior disorders (DBDs) are disorders in which children or teens have trouble controlling their emotions and behavior. Their behavior may be very defiant, and they may strongly conflict with authority figures. Their actions may be aggressive and destructive. All children have mild behavior problems now and then, but the symptoms of DBDs are more severe and continue over time.

Disruptive behavior disorders can start when a child is young. Children or teens with a DBD who do not receive treatment often have serious behavior problems at home, at school, or both. They are also more likely to have problems with alcohol or drug use and violent or criminal behavior as they get older.

DISRUPTIVE MOOD DYSREGULATION DISORDER

Disruptive mood dysregulation disorder (DMDD) is a childhood condition of extreme irritability, anger, and frequent, intense temper outbursts. DMDD symptoms go beyond a being a "moody" child—children with DMDD experience severe impairment that requires clinical attention. DMDD is a fairly new diagnosis, appearing for the first time in the *Diagnostic and Statistical Manual of Mental Disorders* (*DSM-5*), published in 2013.

Disruptive mood dysregulation disorder is a new diagnosis. Therefore, treatment is often based on what has been helpful for other disorders that share the symptoms of irritability and temper tantrums. These disorders include attention deficit hyperactivity disorder (ADHD), anxiety disorders, oppositional defiant disorder, and major depressive disorder.

While researchers are still determining which treatments work best, two major types of treatment are currently used to treat DMDD symptoms:

- Medication
- Psychological treatments
    - Psychotherapy
    - Parent training
    - Computer-based training

Psychological treatments should be considered first, with medication added later if necessary, or psychological treatments can be provided along with medication from the beginning.

EATING DISORDERS

Eating disorders are serious behavior problems. They can include severe overeating or not consuming enough food to stay healthy. They also involve extreme concern about your shape or weight.

Types of eating disorders include:

- Anorexia nervosa, in which you become too thin, but you do not eat enough because you think you are fat
- Bulimia nervosa, which involves periods of overeating followed by purging, sometimes through self-induced vomiting or using laxatives
- Binge-eating, which is out-of-control eating

Women are more likely than men to have eating disorders. They usually start in the teenage years and often occur along with depression, anxiety disorders, and substance abuse.

Eating disorders can lead to heart and kidney problems and even death. Getting help early is important. Treatment involves monitoring, talk therapy, nutritional counseling, and sometimes medicines.

GENERALIZED ANXIETY DISORDER

Occasional anxiety is a normal part of life. You might worry about things like health, money, or family problems. But, people with generalized anxiety disorder (GAD) feel extremely worried or feel nervous about these and other things—even when there is little or no reason to worry about them. People with GAD find it difficult to control their anxiety and stay focused on daily tasks.

GAD is generally treated with psychotherapy, medication, or both. Talk with your doctor about the best treatment for you.

OBSESSIVE-COMPULSIVE DISORDER

Obsessive-compulsive disorder (OCD) is a common, chronic (long-lasting) disorder in which a person has uncontrollable, reoccurring thoughts (obsessions), and behaviors (compulsions) that she or he feels the urge to repeat over and over in response to the obsession.

While everyone sometimes feels the need to double check things, people with OCD have uncontrollable thoughts that cause them anxiety, urging them to check things repeatedly or perform routines and rituals for at least one hour per day. Performing the routines or rituals may bring brief but temporary relief from the anxiety. However, left untreated, these thoughts and rituals cause the person great distress and get in the way of work, school, and personal relationships.

The first step is to talk with your doctor or healthcare provider about your symptoms. The clinician should do an exam and ask you about your health history to make sure that a physical problem is not causing your symptoms. Your doctor may refer you to a mental-health specialist, such as a psychiatrist, psychologist, social worker, or counselor, for further evaluation or treatment.

Obsessive-compulsive disorder is generally treated with cognitive behavior therapy, medication, or both. Speak with your mental-health professional about the best treatment for you.

PERSONALITY DISORDERS

Personality disorders are a group of mental illnesses. They involve long-term patterns of thoughts and behaviors that are unhealthy and inflexible. The behaviors cause serious problems with relationships and work. People with personality disorders have trouble dealing with everyday stresses and problems. They often have stormy relationships with other people.

The cause of personality disorders is unknown. However, genes and childhood experiences may play a role.

The symptoms of each personality disorder are different. They can mild or severe. People with personality disorders may have trouble realizing that they have a problem. To them, their thoughts are normal, and they often blame others for their problems. They may try to get help because of their problems with relationships and work. Treatment usually includes talk therapy and sometimes medicine.

POSTTRAUMATIC STRESS DISORDER

Posttraumatic stress disorder (PTSD) is a real illness. You can get PTSD after living through or seeing a traumatic event, such as war, a hurricane, sexual assault, physical abuse, or a bad accident. PTSD makes you feel stressed and afraid after the danger is over. It affects your life and the people around you.

PTSD can cause problems such as:

- Flashbacks, or feeling like the event is happening again
- Trouble sleeping or nightmares
- Feeling alone
- Angry outbursts
- Feeling worried, guilty, or sad

PTSD starts at different times for different people. Signs of PTSD may start soon after a frightening event and then continue. Other people develop new or more severe signs months or even years later. PTSD can happen to anyone, even children.

Treatment may include talk therapy, medicines, or both. Treatment might take 6 to 12 weeks. For some people, it takes longer.

Chapter 10 | **Common Psychotic Disorders**

Section 10.1 | Delusional Disorder

WHAT IS DELUSIONAL DISORDER?

A delusion is a mistaken impression maintained by an individual that is contradictory to reality or plausible explanation. Persons with delusional disorder (DD) have untrue beliefs that persist for more than a month's duration. Some delusions that patients experience cannot be explained, but some of them could be realistic and lead to the disorder remaining undiagnosed. Delusional disorder, previously known as "paranoid disorder," is classified under psychotic illnesses. People with delusional disorder perceive things differently and misinterpret experiences.

Delusional disorder differs from other psychotic disorders with respect to how people carry on with their daily lives. People with more common psychotic disorders, such as schizophrenia, become so preoccupied with their delusions that it hampers their daily routine. Those with delusional disorder, on the other hand, function normally in society. They remain employed, perform daily tasks without hindrance, and do not act bizarrely. The incidence of delusional disorder in the general population is rare. The disorder occurs in middle to late adulthood and occurs more in women than men.

WHAT ARE THE SYMPTOMS AND SUBTYPES OF DELUSIONAL DISORDER?

The dominant or only symptom of delusional disorder is delusions. While delusions are prominent in other psychotic disorders, such as schizophrenia and bipolar disorder, the absence of accompanying symptoms, such as hallucinations, mood swings, disorganized thinking, and cognitive deficits are used to make the diagnosis of delusional disorder. Early signs of illness may include a basic mistrust of people, unwarranted jealousy of a spouse, or a preoccupation with loyalty in relation to friends and relatives. The person is also overly sensitive to harmless remarks or perceived slights and tends to hold a long-standing grudge toward the subject of their delusion despite evidence to the contrary.

Some of the recognized subtypes of delusional disorder are:

- **Erotomania.** Implausible belief held by the affected person that another person is in love her or him. The person believed to be in love with the delusional person can be a famous person or a total stranger. Those suffering from this type of delusional disorder will often try to establish contact with the object of their fixation through letters, telephone calls, and surveillance. This may be tantamount to stalking and may have legal implications.
- **Jealous type.** Delusional belief that her or his spouse (or sexual partner) is unfaithful. Also known as "conjugal paranoia," or "Othello syndrome," the affected person justifies her or his conviction on the basis of false conclusions despite the lack of objective evidence. Physical violence may or may not accompany this subtype.
- **Grandiose type.** Also called "megalomania," this type is characterized by exaggerated beliefs of grandeur and self-worth as well as extreme arrogance. The affected person believes he or she is omnipotent, famous, and powerful, and the delusions typically have a religious, fictional, or supernatural content.
- **Persecutory.** Persistent conviction that he or she is being plotted against, maligned, or harassed with intent to cause harm. The person with this delusion may relentlessly seek legal recourse through courts and law-enforcement agencies and may even resort to violence in retaliation for the perceived threat.
- **Somatic.** Characterized by an intense preoccupation with imagined defects in physical appearance (body dysmorphic disorder) and bodily function (hypochondriasis), which focuses on imagined illnesses/disorders contrary to medical evidence. This type may also include delusional infestation (DI) in which the affected persons hold a rigid belief that they are infested with parasites or pathogens, and patients may typically describe sensations of "crawling" and "biting" to substantiate their beliefs.

HOW IS DELUSIONAL DISORDER DIAGNOSED?

Delusional disorder is diagnosed on the basis of a thorough psychological assessment. A physical examination and diagnostic tests, including imaging tests and blood tests, are carried out to rule out other causes. Interviews with family members and friends to understand past history and behavioral symptoms are important tools that assist in diagnosis. Nonbizarre delusions persisting for more than a month and absence of symptoms related to schizophrenia and other psychotic disorders lead to confirmation of this diagnosis. The doctor will also assess if the person will likely act on delusions.

WHAT CAUSES DELUSIONAL DISORDER

The causes and triggers for the delusional disorder are not known in medical circles. But the following factors are thought to play a role.

- **Genetics.** The disorder is seen in families that have a history of schizophrenia and delusional disorder, suggesting a genetic link. The disorder might be inherited by children hereditarily.
- **Environmental or psychological.** There is evidence that suggests that the disorder may develop as a result of stress. Substance abuse such as alcoholism and drug abuse could lead to the disorder. Remaining in isolation is also a risk factor. The disorder has been identified in refugees, particularly in people with low sight and hearing, leading to the observation.
- **Biological.** Researchers are investigating anomalies in the brain that could be a contributing factor for the disorder. Defects in regions of the brain that control perception and thinking may be linked to the disorder.

WHAT IS THE TREATMENT FOR DELUSIONAL DISORDER?

A combination of psychotherapy and medication is used to treat delusional disorder. Denial about delusions, poor insight, and refusal to seek help are deterrents to treatment. Establishing a good rapport between doctor and patient is crucial to successful treatment. Medications help in recovery to some extent. Medications commonly used for treatment include conventional antipsychotics (neuroleptics), atypical antipsychotics, tranquilizers, and antidepressants. Psychotherapy is also recommended and therapy types such as cognitive behavior therapy, family therapy, and individual counseling help the person manage stress and the impact of delusions in daily functioning.

WHAT ARE THE COMPLICATIONS THAT ARISE DUE TO DELUSIONAL DISORDER?

Delusions could lead to depression because of difficulties that arise out of such thinking. Persons who act on their delusions may become violent and get into legal difficulties. If the delusions are severe, then people could become alienated from family and friends.

WHAT IS THE OUTLOOK FOR RECOVERY?

The outlook for recovery depends on factors, such as the type of delusional disorder, life circumstances, what support is available for the person, and her or his willingness to remain under treatment. Delusional disorder is a chronic condition with chances of complete recovery. Some patients experience periods that are free of incidents mixed with episodes of delusions. Most patients with delusional disorder do not seek help because of fear or embarrassment. If treatment is not sought, delusional disorder becomes a lifelong affliction.

IS DELUSIONAL DISORDER PREVENTABLE?

Prevention strategies do not exist currently for delusional disorder but the effect of illness can be minimized with treatment, and the patient can lead a productive life in the company of family and friends.

References

1. "Delusional Disorder and Substance Abuse," American Addiction Centers (AAC), June 17, 2019.
2. "Treatments for Delusional Disorder," Cochrane, May 22, 2015.
3. "Delusional Disorder as a Partial Psychosis," U.S. National Library of Medicine (NLM), 2014.

4. "Understanding Delusions," U.S. National Library of Medicine (NLM), 2009.
5. Schulz, Charles. "Delusional Disorder," Merck Manual, n.d.
6. "Mental Health and Delusional Disorder," WebMD, n.d.

Section 10.2 | Factitious Disorders

"Factitious Disorders," © 2017 Omnigraphics. Reviewed October 2019.

WHAT ARE FACTITIOUS DISORDERS?

Difficult to diagnose and treat, factitious disorder is a rare mental disorder in which an individual acts as though they are sick when in reality they are mimicking or intentionally creating the symptoms of a disease or condition. Patients with factitious disorder may lie about symptoms, bring about symptoms by self-injury, needlessly undergo painful diagnostic procedures, and tamper with the results of the medical tests. Unlike those who lie about medical conditions for monetary gain or other compensation, the only goal of those with factitious disorder is to receive sympathy and special attention from family, friends, and the medical community. Factitious disorder is found to be associated with preexisting mental illnesses such as depression and anxiety as well as stressful living conditions.

Factitious disorder can be subdivided into two types. The first is, referred to as "factitious disorder imposed on self" (In the past this subtype was referred to as "Munchausen syndrome" after the 18th-century German figure who regularly exaggerated his maladies.) The person affected will themselves mimic a mental or physical illness. For example, the person will appear confused, making absurd statements, and say they are hallucinating. They may also bring about physical symptoms such as stomach pains or seizures. The second type is "factitious disorder imposed on others" (previously referred to as "Munchausen by proxy"). In this manifestation, the person will impose false physical or psychological symptoms on another person. This is usually seen with a parent falsely presenting their child as sick, often putting the child at serious risk of harm as the result of unnecessary tests or medical procedures.

WHAT ARE THE SYMPTOMS OF FACTITIOUS DISORDER?

The symptoms of factitious disorder are difficult to pick out as the person can go to great lengths to hide their deception. Warning signs usually involve mimicking or exaggerating sickness or injury as well as:

- Episodes of lying
- Self-injury—Individuals may inject themselves with harmful bacteria, milk, or feces to bring about symptoms or physically injure themselves by cutting or burning
- Tampering with the results of diagnostic tests by such actions as manipulating medical instruments or contaminating urine samples with blood
- Using aliases in order to visit a range of medical facilities and doctors
- Persistent symptoms even after appropriate treatment
- Extensive and specialized knowledge of medical conditions, tests, and treatment procedures
- Repeated hospital stays
- Unwillingness to allow healthcare professionals to talk to their family and friends
- Unwillingness to submit to psychiatric evaluation

WHAT ARE THE CAUSES OF FACTITIOUS DISORDER?

The cause of factitious disorder is unknown, but researchers have found a strong link to preexisting behavioral and psychological issues along with stressful living conditions.

There may be several possible risk factors associated with factitious disorder. Research suggests that a childhood trauma in the form of physical, verbal, or emotional abuse as well as neglect can be a major factor. This can lead to poor sense of self or a loss of identity. Loss of a loved one that leads to a persistent sense of abandonment can also be a factor as well as past experiences of hospital stays that attracted significant attention from family and others. This condition can occasionally be seen in healthcare workers.

DIAGNOSIS OF FACTITIOUS DISORDER

Diagnosing factitious disorder is challenging, given the amount of misinformation provided by the patient. Medical professionals first must gather as much of an accurate medical history as possible despite the exaggerations, misdirection, and potential use of aliases during treatment. They must then also rule out any possible physical or alternate mental condition (such as psychosis), which requires a thorough review of medical tests, imagery, and lab work. Interviewing the patient and observing her or his behavior is also key to diagnosing the condition. The patient may overdramatize her or his symptoms, may present information that contradicts previous medical findings or the recollections of their caregivers, and may appear overeager to submit to painful or invasive tests. Medical professionals will then compare their findings to the criteria for factitious disorder as outlined in *Diagnostic and Statistical Manual of Mental Disorder, Fifth Edition* (*DSM-5*), published by the American Psychiatric Association (APA).

TREATMENT OF FACTITIOUS DISORDER

No standard protocols or therapies are currently available for treatment of factitious disorders. However, it has been found that the affected person will respond better to a nonjudgmental approach. With this kind of approach, they may be more willing to be treated by a mental-health professional. Also, having a primary-care physician or other medical professional act as a gatekeeper who monitors all medical care of a patient is the key to accomplishing the first goal of treatment, which is to end or reduce that person's misuse of the medical system.

Psychotherapy will help in coping with underlying issues, including stress and depression. Medications for preexisting mental-health disorders may be used. If the disorder is found to be serious, extensive hospital stay and treatment may be required.

References

1. "An Overview of Factitious Disorders," Cleveland Clinic, March 28, 2017.
2. "Factitious Disorder," Mayo Clinic, May 31, 2017.

Section 10.3 | Psychosis

This section includes text excerpted from "RAISE Questions and Answers," National Institute of Mental Health (NIMH), October 7, 2015. Reviewed October 2019.

WHAT IS PSYCHOSIS?

The word "psychosis" is used to describe conditions that affect the mind, where there has been some loss of contact with reality. When someone becomes ill in this way, it is called a "psychotic episode." During a period of psychosis, a person's thoughts and perceptions are disturbed and the individual may have difficulty understanding what is real and what is not. Symptoms of psychosis include delusions (false beliefs) and hallucinations (seeing or hearing things that others do not see or hear). Other symptoms include incoherent speech and behavior that is inappropriate for the situation. A person in a psychotic episode may also experience depression, anxiety, sleep problems, social withdrawal, lack of motivation, and difficulty functioning overall.

WHAT CAUSES PSYCHOSIS

There is no one specific cause of psychosis. Psychosis may be a symptom of mental illness, such as schizophrenia or bipolar disorder, but there are other causes as well. Sleep deprivation, some general medical conditions, certain prescription medications, and the abuse of alcohol or other drugs, such as marijuana, can cause psychotic symptoms. Because there are many different causes of psychosis, it is important to see a qualified healthcare professional (e.g., psychologist, psychiatrist, or trained social worker) in order to receive a thorough assessment and accurate diagnosis. A mental illness, such as schizophrenia, is typically diagnosed by excluding all of these other causes of psychosis.

HOW COMMON IS PSYCHOSIS

Approximately 3 percent of the people in the United States (3 out of 100 people) will experience psychosis at some time in their lives.

About 100,000 adolescents and young adults in the United States experience first-episode psychosis each year.

WHAT IS THE CONNECTION BETWEEN PSYCHOSIS AND SCHIZOPHRENIA?

Schizophrenia is a mental illness characterized by periods of psychosis. An individual must experience psychotic symptoms for at least six months in order to be diagnosed with schizophrenia. However, a person may experience psychosis and never be diagnosed with schizophrenia or any other mental-health condition. This is because there are many different causes of psychosis, such as sleep deprivation, general medical conditions, the use of certain prescription medications, and the abuse of alcohol or other drugs.

WHAT ARE THE EARLY WARNING SIGNS OF PSYCHOSIS?

Typically, a person will show changes in their behavior before psychosis develops. The list below includes behavioral warning signs for psychosis:

- A worrisome drop in grades or job performance
- New trouble thinking clearly or concentrating
- Suspiciousness, paranoid ideas, or uneasiness with others
- Withdrawing socially, spending a lot more time alone than usual
- Unusual, overly intense new ideas, strange feelings, or having no feelings at all
- A decline in self-care or personal hygiene
- Difficulty telling reality from fantasy
- Confused speech or trouble communicating

Any one of these items itself may not be significant, but someone with several of the items on the list should consult a mental-health professional. A qualified psychologist, psychiatrist, or trained social worker will be able to make a diagnosis and help develop a treatment plan. Early treatment of psychosis increases the chance of a successful recovery. If you notice these changes in behavior and they begin to intensify or do not go away, it is important to seek help.

WHAT DOES "DURATION OF UNTREATED PSYCHOSIS" MEAN?

The length of time between the start of psychotic symptoms and the beginning of treatment is called the "duration of untreated psychosis," or DUP. In general, research has shown that treatments for psychosis work better when they are delivered closer to the time when symptoms first appear. This was the case in the Recovery After an Initial Schizophrenia Episode-Early Treatment Program (RAISE-ETP) study. Individuals who had a shorter DUP when they started treatment showed much greater improvement in symptoms, functioning, and quality of life than those with longer DUP. The RAISE-ETP project also found that average DUP in the United States is typically longer than what is considered acceptable by international standards. Future RAISE-related efforts are working to find ways of decreasing DUP so that individuals receive care as early as possible after symptoms appear.

DO PEOPLE RECOVER FROM PSYCHOSIS?

With early diagnosis and appropriate treatment, it is possible to recover from psychosis. Many people who receive early treatment never have another psychotic episode. For other people, recovery means the ability to live a fulfilling and productive life, even if psychotic symptoms return sometimes.

WHAT SHOULD I DO IF I THINK SOMEONE IS HAVING A PSYCHOTIC EPISODE?

If you think someone you know is experiencing psychosis, encourage the person to seek treatment as early as possible. Psychosis can be treated effectively, and early intervention increases the chance of a successful outcome. To find a qualified treatment program, contact your healthcare professional. If someone having a psychotic episode is in distress or you are concerned about their safety, consider taking them to the nearest emergency room, or call 911.

Section 10.4 | Schizoaffective Disorder

This section includes text excerpted from "Facts about Schizoaffective Disorder," Mental Illness Research, Education and Clinical Centers (MIRECC), U.S. Department of Veterans Affairs (VA), November 20, 2013. Reviewed October 2019.

WHAT IS SCHIZOAFFECTIVE DISORDER?

Schizoaffective disorder is a major psychiatric disorder that is quite similar to schizophrenia. The disorder can affect all aspects of daily living, including work, social relationships, and self-care skills (such as grooming and hygiene). People with schizoaffective disorder can have a wide variety of different symptoms, including having unusual perceptual experiences (hallucinations) or beliefs others do not share (delusions), mood (such as marked depression), low motivation, inability to experience pleasure, and poor attention. The serious nature of the symptoms of schizoaffective disorder sometimes requires people to go to the hospital for care. The experience of schizoaffective disorder can be described as similar to "dreaming when you are wide awake"; that is, it can be hard for the person with the disorder to distinguish between reality and fantasy.

HOW COMMON IS SCHIZOAFFECTIVE DISORDER?

About one in every two hundred people (0.5%) develops schizoaffective disorder at some time during her or his life. Schizoaffective disorder, along with schizophrenia, is one of the most common serious psychiatric disorders. More hospital beds are occupied by persons with these disorders than any other psychiatric disorder. However, as with other types of mental illness, individuals with schizoaffective disorder can engage in treatment and other mental-health recovery efforts that have the potential to dramatically improve the well-being of the individual.

HOW IS THE DISORDER DIAGNOSED?

Schizoaffective disorder can only be diagnosed by a clinical interview. The purpose of the interview is to determine whether the person has experienced specific "symptoms" of the disorder and whether these symptoms have been present long enough to merit the diagnosis. In addition to conducting the interview, the diagnostician must also check to make sure the person is not experiencing any physical problems that could cause symptoms similar to schizoaffective disorder, such as a brain tumor or alcohol or drug abuse.

Schizoaffective disorder cannot be diagnosed with a blood test, x-ray, computerized axial tomography (CAT) scan, or any other laboratory test. An interview is necessary to establish the diagnosis.

CHARACTERISTIC SYMPTOMS OF SCHIZOAFFECTIVE DISORDER

The diagnosis of schizoaffective disorder requires that the person experience some decline in social functioning for at least a six-month period, such as problems with school or work, social relationships, or self-care. In addition, some other symptoms must be commonly present. The symptoms of schizoaffective disorder can be divided into five broad classes: positive symptoms, negative symptoms, symptoms of mania, symptoms of depression, and other symptoms. A person with schizoaffective disorder will usually have some (but not all) of the symptoms described below.

POSITIVE SYMPTOMS OF SCHIZOAFFECTIVE DISORDER

Positive symptoms refer to thoughts, perceptions, and behaviors that are ordinarily absent in persons who are not diagnosed with schizophrenia or schizoaffective disorder but are present in persons with schizoaffective disorder. These symptoms often vary over time in their severity and may be absent for long periods in some persons.

Hallucinations. Hallucinations are "false perceptions"; that is, hearing, seeing, feeling, or smelling things that are not actually there. The most common type of hallucination is auditory hallucinations. Individuals sometimes report hearing voices talking to them or about them, often saying insulting things, such as calling them names. These voices are usually heard through the ears and sound like other human voices.

Delusions. Delusions are "false beliefs"; that is, a belief which the person holds, but which others do not share. Some individuals have paranoid delusions, believing that they are not safe or others want to hurt them. Delusions of reference are common, in which the individual believes that something in the environment is referring to her or him when it is not (such as the television talking to the person). Delusions of control are beliefs that others can control one's actions. Individuals may hold these beliefs strongly and cannot usually be "talked out" of them.

Thinking disturbances. This problem is reflected in a difficulty in communication. The individual talks in a manner that is difficult to follow. For example, the individual may jump from one topic to the next, stop in the middle of the sentence, make up new words, or simply be difficult to understand.

NEGATIVE SYMPTOMS OF SCHIZOAFFECTIVE DISORDER

Negative symptoms are the opposite of positive symptoms. They are the absence of thoughts, perceptions, or behaviors that are ordinarily present in people who are not diagnosed with schizophrenia or schizoaffective disorder. These symptoms can often persist for a long period of time, though with effort on the individual's part they can often be improved. Many professionals think these symptoms reflect a sense of hopelessness about the future.

Blunted affect. The expressiveness of the individual's face, voice tone, and gestures is less. However, this does not mean that the person is not reacting to her or his environment or having feelings.

Apathy. The individual does not feel motivated to pursue goals and activities. The individual may feel lethargic or sleepy and have trouble following through on even simple plans. Individuals with apathy often have little sense of purpose in their lives and have few interests.

Anhedonia. The individual experiences little or no pleasure from activities that she or he used to enjoy or that others enjoy. For example, the person may not enjoy watching a sunset, going to the movies, or a close relationship with another person.

Poverty of speech or content of speech. The individual says very little, or when she or he talks, there does not seem to be much information being conveyed. Sometimes conversing with the person with schizoaffective disorder can be very difficult.

Inattention. The individual has difficulty paying attention and is easily distracted. This can interfere with activities such as work, interacting with others, and personal-care skills.

SYMPTOMS OF MANIA

In general, the symptoms of mania involve an excess in behavioral activity, mood states (in particular, irritability or positive feelings), and self-esteem and confidence.

- **Euphoric or expansive mood.** The individual's mood is abnormally elevated, such as extremely happy or excited (euphoria). The person may tend to talk more and with greater enthusiasm or emphasis on certain topics (expansiveness).
- **Irritability.** The individual is easily angered or persistently irritable, especially when others seem to interfere with her or his plans or goals, however, unrealistic they may be.
- **Inflated self-esteem or grandiosity.** The individual is extremely self-confident and maybe unrealistic about her or his abilities (grandiosity). For example, the individual may believe she or he is a brilliant artist or inventor, a wealthy person, a shrewd businessperson, or a healer when she or he has no special competence in these areas.
- **Decreased need for sleep.** Only a few hours of sleep are needed each night (such as less than four hours) for the individual to feel rested.
- **Talkativeness.** The individual talks excessively and may be difficult to interrupt. The individual may jump quickly from one topic to another (called "flight of ideas"), making it hard for others to understand.
- **Racing thoughts.** Thoughts come so rapidly that the individual finds it hard to keep up with them or express them.
- **Distractibility.** The individual's attention is easily drawn to irrelevant stimuli, such as the sound of a car honking outside on the street.
- **Increased goal-directed activity.** A great deal of time is spent pursuing specific goals, at work, school, or sexually. Often these behaviors put the person at risk.

- **Excessive involvement in pleasurable activities with high potential for negative consequences.** Common problem areas include spending sprees, sexual indiscretions, increased substance abuse, or making foolish business investments.

SYMPTOMS OF DEPRESSION

Depressive symptoms reflect the opposite end of the continuum of mood from manic symptoms, with a low mood and behavioral inactivity as the major features.

Depressed mood. The mood is low most of the time, according to the person or significant others.

Diminished interest or pleasure. The individual has few interests and gets little pleasure from anything, including activities previously found enjoyable.

Change in appetite and/or weight. Loss of appetite (and weight) when not dieting, or increased appetite (and weight gain) are evident.

Change in sleep pattern. The individual may have difficulty falling asleep, staying asleep, or wake early in the morning and not be able to get back to sleep. Alternatively, the person may sleep excessively (such as over twelve hours per night), spending much of the day in bed.

Change in activity level. Decreased activity level is reflected by slowness and lethargy, both in terms of the individual's behavior and thought processes. Alternatively, the individual may feel agitated, "on edge," and restless.

Fatigue or loss of energy. The individual experiences fatigue throughout the day or there is a chronic feeling of loss of energy.

Feelings of worthlessness, hopelessness, helplessness. Individuals may feel they are worthless as people, that there is no hope for improving their lives, or that there is no point in trying to improve their unhappy situation.

Inappropriate guilt. Feelings of guilt may be present about events that the individual did not even do, such as a catastrophe, a crime, or an illness.

Recurrent thoughts about death. The individual thinks about death a great deal and may contemplate (or even attempt) suicide.

Decreased concentration or ability to make decisions. Significant decreases in the ability to concentrate make it difficult for the individual to pay attention to others or complete simple tasks. The individual may be quite indecisive about even minor things.

OTHER SYMPTOMS

Individuals with schizoaffective disorder are prone to alcohol or drug abuse. Some individuals may use alcohol and drugs excessively either because of their disturbing symptoms, to experience pleasure, or when socializing with others.

HOW IS SCHIZOAFFECTIVE DISORDER DISTINGUISHED FROM SCHIZOPHRENIA AND AFFECTIVE (MOOD) DISORDERS?

Many persons with a diagnosis of schizoaffective disorder have had, at a prior time, diagnoses of schizophrenia or bipolar disorder. Frequently, this previous diagnosis is revised to schizoaffective disorder when it becomes clear, over time, that the person experiences symptoms of mania or depression much of the time, but on other occasions have experienced psychotic symptoms, such as hallucinations or delusions even when her or his mood is stable.

WHAT IS THE COURSE OF SCHIZOAFFECTIVE DISORDER?

The disorder usually begins in late adolescence or early adulthood, often between the ages of sixteen and thirty. The severity of symptoms usually varies over time, at times requiring hospitalization for treatment. The disorder is often life-long, although the symptoms tend to improve gradually over the person's life and many individuals who were diagnosed with the disorder when they were younger appear to have few or no symptoms from middle age on. With schizoaffective disorder, as with other major psychiatric illnesses, individuals can work to achieve their goals and live very full lives.

WHAT CAUSES SCHIZOAFFECTIVE DISORDER

The cause of schizoaffective disorder is not known, although many scientists believe it is a variant of the disorder of schizophrenia.

Schizoaffective disorder (and schizophrenia) may actually be several disorders. Current theories suggest that an imbalance in brain chemicals (specifically, dopamine) may be at the root of these two disorders. Vulnerability to developing schizoaffective disorder appears to be partly determined by genetic factors and partly by early environmental factors (such as subtle insults to the brain of the baby in the womb before and during birth).

HOW IS SCHIZOAFFECTIVE DISORDER TREATED?

Many of the same methods used to treat schizophrenia are also effective for schizoaffective disorder. Antipsychotic medications are an effective treatment for schizoaffective disorder for most, but not all, persons with the disorder. These drugs are not a "cure" for the disorder, but they can reduce symptoms and prevent relapses among the majority of people with the disorder. Antidepressant medications and mood-stabilizing medications (such as lithium) are occasionally used to treat affective symptoms (depressive or manic symptoms) in schizoaffective disorder. Other important treatments include social skills training, vocational rehabilitation and supported employment, peer support, and intensive case management. Family therapy helps reduce stress in the family and teaches family members how to monitor the disorder. In addition, individual supportive counseling can help the person with the disorder learn to manage the disorder more successfully and obtain emotional support in coping with the distress resulting from the disorder. Individuals with schizoaffective disorder who work actively toward mental-health recovery can positively affect the course of their illness and improve the quality of their lives. Family support for the individual's recovery efforts can lend meaningful benefits.

Section 10.5 | **Schizophrenia**

This section includes text excerpted from "Schizophrenia," National Institute of Mental Health (NIMH), February 15, 2016. Reviewed October 2019.

WHAT IS SCHIZOPHRENIA?

Schizophrenia is a chronic and severe mental disorder that affects how a person thinks, feels, and behaves. People with schizophrenia may seem like they have lost touch with reality. Although schizophrenia is not as common as other mental disorders, the symptoms can be very disabling.

SIGNS AND SYMPTOMS OF SCHIZOPHRENIA

Symptoms of schizophrenia usually start between ages 16 and 30. In rare cases, children have schizophrenia too.

The symptoms of schizophrenia fall into three categories: positive, negative, and cognitive.

Positive symptoms. "Positive" symptoms are psychotic behaviors not generally seen in healthy people. People with positive symptoms may "lose touch" with some aspects of reality. Symptoms include:

- Hallucinations
- Delusions
- Thought disorders (unusual or dysfunctional ways of thinking)
- Movement disorders (agitated body movements)

Negative symptoms. "Negative" symptoms are associated with disruptions to normal emotions and behaviors. Symptoms include:

- "Flat affect" (reduced expression of emotions via facial expression or voice tone)
- Reduced feelings of pleasure in everyday life
- Difficulty beginning and sustaining activities
- Reduced speaking

Cognitive symptoms. For some patients, the cognitive symptoms of schizophrenia are subtle, but for others, they are more severe and patients may notice changes in their memory or other aspects of thinking. Symptoms include:

- Poor "executive functioning" (the ability to understand information and use it to make decisions)
- Trouble focusing or paying attention
- Challenges involving "working memory" (the ability to use the information immediately after learning it)

RISK FACTORS OF SCHIZOPHRENIA

There are several factors that contribute to the risk of developing schizophrenia.

Genes and environment. Scientists have long known that schizophrenia sometimes runs in families. However, there are many people who have schizophrenia who do not have a family member with the disorder and conversely, many people with one or more family members with the disorder do not develop it themselves.

Scientists believe that many different genes may increase the risk of schizophrenia, but that no single gene causes the disorder by itself. It is not yet possible to use genetic information to predict who will develop schizophrenia.

Scientists also think that interactions between genes and aspects of the individual's environment are necessary for schizophrenia to develop. Environmental factors may involve:

- Exposure to viruses
- Malnutrition before birth
- Problems during birth
- Psychosocial factors

Different brain chemistry and structure. Scientists think that an imbalance in the complex, interrelated chemical reactions of the brain involving the neurotransmitters (substances that brain cells use to communicate with each other) dopamine and glutamate, and possibly others, plays a role in schizophrenia.

Some experts also think problems during brain development before birth may lead to faulty connections. The brain also undergoes major changes during puberty, and these changes could trigger psychotic symptoms in people who are vulnerable due to genetics or brain differences.

TREATMENTS AND THERAPIES OF SCHIZOPHRENIA

Because the causes of schizophrenia are still unknown, treatments focus on eliminating the symptoms of the disease. Treatments include:

Antipsychotics

Antipsychotic medications are usually taken daily in pill or liquid form. Some antipsychotics are injections that are given once or twice a month. Some people have side effects when they start taking medications, but most side effects go away after a few days. Doctors and patients can work together to find the best medication or medication combination, and the right dose.

Psychosocial Treatments

These treatments are helpful after patients and their doctor finds a medication that works. Learning and using coping skills to address the everyday challenges of schizophrenia helps people to pursue their life goals, such as attending school or work. Individuals who participate in regular psychosocial treatment are less likely to have relapses or be hospitalized.

Coordinated Specialty Care

This treatment model integrates medication, psychosocial therapies, case management, family involvement, and supported education and employment services, all aimed at reducing symptoms and improving quality of life. The National Institute of Mental Health (NIMH) Recovery After an Initial Schizophrenia Episode (RAISE) research project seeks to fundamentally change the trajectory and prognosis of schizophrenia through coordinated specialty care treatment in the earliest stages of the disorder. RAISE is designed to reduce the likelihood of long-term disability that people with schizophrenia often experience and help them lead productive, independent lives.

How Can I Help Someone I Know with Schizophrenia?

Caring for and supporting a loved one with schizophrenia can be hard. It can be difficult to know how to respond to someone who makes strange or clearly false statements. It is important to understand that schizophrenia is a biological illness.

Here are some things you can do to help your loved one:

- Get them to treatment and encourage them to stay in treatment
- Remember that their beliefs or hallucinations seem very real to them
- Tell them that you acknowledge that everyone has the right to see things their own way
- Be respectful, supportive, and kind without tolerating dangerous or inappropriate behavior
- Check to see if there are any support groups in your area

Part 2 | **Personal, Social, and Economic Impact of Mental Disability**

Chapter 11 | How Does a Mental Disability Affect a Person's Life?

OVERVIEW AND IMPACT

The burden of mental illness in the United States is among the highest of all diseases and mental disorders are among the most common causes of disability. Data suggest that, in 2004, approximately 1 in 4 adults in the United States had a mental-health disorder in the past year—most commonly anxiety or depression—and 1 in 17 had a serious mental illness. Mental-health disorders also affect children and adolescents at an increasingly alarming rate; in 2010, 1 in 5 children in the United States had a mental-health disorder, most commonly attention deficit hyperactivity disorder (ADHD). It is not unusual for either adults or children to have more than one mental-health disorder.

Mental health is essential to a person's well-being, healthy family and interpersonal relationships, and the ability to live a full and productive life. People, including children and adolescents, with untreated mental-health disorders, are at high risk for many unhealthy and unsafe behaviors, including alcohol or drug abuse, violent or self-destructive behavior, and suicide—the 11th leading cause of death in the United States for all age groups and the second leading cause of death among people age 25 to 34.

This chapter contains text excerpted from the following sources: Text beginning with the heading "Overview and Impact" is excerpted from "Mental Health," Office of Disease Prevention and Health Promotion (ODPHP), U.S. Department of Health and Human Services (HHS), October 31, 2011. Reviewed October 2019; Text under the heading "Life Expectancy and Mental Illness" is excerpted from "Post by Former NIMH Director Thomas Insel: No Health without Mental Health," National Institute of Mental Health (NIMH), September 6, 2011. Reviewed October 2019.

Mental-health disorders also have a serious impact on physical health and are associated with the prevalence, progression, and outcome of some of today's most pressing chronic diseases, including diabetes, heart disease, and cancer. Mental-health disorders can have harmful and long-lasting effects—including high psychosocial and economic costs—not only for people living with the disorder, but also for their families, schools, workplaces, and communities.

Fortunately, a number of mental-health disorders can be treated effectively, and the prevention of mental-health disorders is a growing area of research and practice. Early diagnosis and treatment can decrease the disease burden of mental-health disorders as well as associated chronic diseases. Assessing and addressing mental health remains important to ensure that all Americans lead longer, healthier lives.

Health Impact of Mental Health

Mental health and physical health are inextricably linked. Evidence has shown that mental-health disorders—most often depression—are strongly associated with the risk, occurrence, management, progression, and outcome of serious chronic diseases and health conditions, including diabetes, hypertension, stroke, heart disease, and cancer. This association appears to be caused by mental-health disorders that precede chronic disease; the chronic disease can intensify the symptoms of mental-health disorders—in effect creating a cycle of poor health. This cycle decreases a person's ability to participate in the treatment of and recovery from mental-health disorders and chronic disease. Therefore, while efforts are underway to reduce the burden of death and disability caused by chronic disease in the United States, simultaneously improving mental health nationwide is critical to improving the health of all Americans.

MENTAL HEALTH ACROSS THE LIFE STAGES

Mental-health disorders are a concern for people of all ages, from early childhood through old age.

Children and Adolescents

- Approximately, 20 percent of U.S. children and adolescents are affected by mental-health disorders during their lifetime. Often, symptoms of anxiety disorders emerge by age 6,

behavior disorders by age 11, mood disorders by age 13, and substance-use disorders (SUDs) by age 15.
- 15 percent of high-school students have seriously considered suicide, and 7 percent have attempted to take their own life.
- Mental-health disorders among children and adolescents can lead to school failure, alcohol or other drug abuse, family discord, violence, and suicide.

Adults

- It is estimated that only about 17 percent of U.S. adults are considered to be in a state of optimal mental health.
- An estimated 26 percent of Americans age 18 and older are living with a mental-health disorder in any given year, and 46 percent will have a mental-health disorder over the course of their lifetime.
- Almost 15 percent of women who gave birth reported symptoms of postpartum depression.

Older Adults

- Alzheimer disease (AD) is among the 10 leading causes of death in the United States. It is the 6th leading cause of death among American adults and the 5th leading cause of death for adults age 65 years and older.
- Among nursing home residents, 18.7 percent of people age 65 to 74 and 23.5 percent of people aged 85 and older have reported the mental illness.

LIFE EXPECTANCY AND MENTAL ILLNESS

Five years ago, Colton and Mandersheidi surveyed mortality data from eight states and concluded that, on average, Americans with major mental illness die 14 to 32 years earlier than the general population. The average life expectancy for people with major mental illness ranged from 49 to 60 years of age in the states they examined—a life span on par with many sub-Saharan African countries, including Sudan (58.6 years) and Ethiopia (52.9 years). The average life expectancy in the United States is 77.9 years. It would appear that the increase in longevity enjoyed by the general U.S. population over the past half-century has been lost on those with serious mental illness (SMI). In fact, this drop in life expectancy due to mental illness would surpass the health disparities reported for most racial or ethnic groups. Yet this population is rarely identified as an underserved or at-risk group in surveys of the social determinants of health.

Chapter 12 | Common Barriers to Participation

Nearly everyone faces hardships and difficulties at one time or another. But, for people with disabilities, barriers can be more frequent and have a greater impact. The World Health Organization (WHO) describes barriers as being more than just physical obstacles. Here is the WHO definition of barriers:

> Factors in a person's environment that, through their absence or presence, limit functioning and create disability. These include aspects such as:
> - A physical environment that is not accessible
> - Lack of relevant assistive technology (assistive, adaptive, and rehabilitative devices)
> - Negative attitudes of people towards disability
> - Services, systems, and policies that are either nonexistent or that hinder the involvement of all people with a health condition in all areas of life.

Often there are multiple barriers that can make it extremely difficult or even impossible for people with disabilities to function. Here are the seven most common barriers. Often, more than one barrier occurs at a time.

- Attitudinal
- Communication
- Physical
- Policy
- Programmatic

This chapter includes text excerpted from "Common Barriers to Participation Experienced by People with Disabilities," Centers for Disease Control and Prevention (CDC), September 4, 2019.

- Social
- Transportation

ATTITUDINAL BARRIERS

Attitudinal barriers are the most basic and contribute to other barriers. For example, some people may not be aware that difficulties in getting to or into a place can limit a person with a disability from participating in everyday life and common daily activities. Examples of attitudinal barriers include:

- **Stereotyping.** People sometimes stereotype those with disabilities, assuming their quality of life is poor or that they are unhealthy because of their impairments.
- **Stigma, prejudice, and discrimination.** Within society, these attitudes may come from people's ideas related to disability—People may see disability as a personal tragedy, as something that needs to be cured or prevented, as a punishment for wrongdoing, or as an indication of the lack of ability to behave as expected in society.

Today, society's understanding of disability is improving as we recognize "disability" as what occurs when a person's functional needs are not addressed in her or his physical and social environment. By not considering disability a personal deficit or shortcoming, and instead of thinking of it as a social responsibility in which all people can be supported to live independent and full lives, it becomes easier to recognize and address challenges that all people—including those with disabilities—experience.

COMMUNICATION BARRIERS

Communication barriers are experienced by people who have disabilities that affect hearing, speaking, reading, writing, and or understanding, and who use different ways to communicate than people who do not have these disabilities. Examples of communication barriers include:

- Written health promotion messages with barriers that prevent people with vision impairments from receiving the message. These include:

    - Use of small print or no large-print versions of the material, and
    - No Braille or versions for people who use screen readers.
- Auditory health messages may be inaccessible to people with hearing impairments, including:
    - Videos that do not include captioning, and
    - Oral communications without accompanying manual interpretation (such as American Sign Language (ASL)).
- The use of technical language, long sentences, and words with many syllables may be significant barriers to understanding for people with cognitive impairments.

POLICY BARRIERS

Policy barriers are frequently related to a lack of awareness or enforcement of existing laws and regulations that require programs and activities to be accessible to people with disabilities. Examples of policy barriers include:

- Denying qualified individuals with disabilities the opportunity to participate in or benefit from federally funded programs, services, or other benefits
- Denying individuals with disabilities access to programs, services, benefits, or opportunities to participate as a result of physical barriers and
- Denying reasonable accommodations to qualified individuals with disabilities, so they can perform the essential functions of the job for which they have applied or have been hired to perform

PROGRAMMATIC BARRIERS

Programmatic barriers limit the effective delivery of a public health or healthcare program for people with different types of impairments. Examples of programmatic barriers include:

- Inconvenient scheduling
- Lack of accessible equipment (such as mammography screening equipment)
- Insufficient time set aside for medical examination and procedures

- Little or no communication with patients or participants
- Provider's attitudes, knowledge, and understanding of people with disabilities

SOCIAL BARRIERS

Social barriers are related to the conditions in which people are born, grow, live, learn, work and age—or social determinants of health—that can contribute to decreased functioning among people with disabilities. Here are examples of social barriers:

- People with disabilities are far less likely to be employed. The unemployment rate in 2012 for people with disabilities was more than 1 in 10 (13.9%) compared to less than 1 in 10 (6.0%) for those without disabilities.
- Adults age 25 years and older with disabilities are less likely to have completed high school compared to their peers without disabilities (23.5% compared to 11.1%).
- People with disabilities are more likely to live in poverty compared to people without disabilities (21.6% compared to 12.8%).
- Children with disabilities are almost four times more likely to experience violence than children without disabilities.

TRANSPORTATION BARRIERS

Transportation barriers are due to a lack of adequate transportation that interferes with a person's ability to be independent and to function in society. Examples of transportation barriers include:

- Lack of access to accessible or convenient transportation for people who are not able to drive because of vision or cognitive impairments, and
- Public transportation may be unavailable or at inconvenient distances or locations.

Chapter 13 | Impact of Disability on Family and Interpersonal Relationships

It is well known that mental illness is a common condition around the world. One in five people experience mental illness at some point in their lives and the most common of these illnesses are depression and anxiety. In addition, at least two to three percent of adults will experience a more serious type of mental disability, such as schizophrenia or bipolar disorder, at some point in their lives.

The effects that mental illness has on one's family and relationships are significant and professional help and support may be required in order to improve outcomes for a person experiencing mental illness.

THE INTERPERSONAL NATURE OF MENTAL-HEALTH DISORDERS

Mental-health disorders are experienced at a personal level and are not generally shared with others. Individuals experiencing adverse mental-health symptoms tend to hide or downplay the seriousness of their difficulties. The extent of their disorder may only be discovered by observing their behaviors closely and recognizing the potential harm being caused by their symptoms.

However, mental disability is also interpersonal. In many cases, the most common symptoms or behaviors exhibited by an individual experiencing mental illness are notable anxiety and difficulty maintaining a social life. Though it can be hard for some family members to recognize the illness, it is generally a close family member or friend who first recognizes that a loved one is acting differently and encourages their loved one to seek immediate help and support.

Interpersonal difficulties may also arise among those in occupational roles, such as parenting, when mental disability is present. Postnatal depression is one example, since people who are parenting while experiencing this mental-health issue may find it hard to develop an attachment toward their child.

Another interpersonal feature is the social stigma that can negatively influence a person with a mental-health disorder. Similarly, self-stigma may lead some individuals to harm themselves.

Both types of stigma are associated with a reluctance to seek help for a mental-health condition. The individual may be especially sensitive to the opinions or presumptions of others, and this, in turn, can affect their willingness to talk about their problems or seek professional help.

IMPACT ON FAMILIES

Research suggests that caregiving for a person who is mentally disabled can also lead to caregiver distress as individuals in this role struggle to cope with perceived judgments and social responses to the mental illness. Researchers have identified a connection between caregiver anxiety and emotional over involvement with a person being treated for mental illness.

For example, in the case of schizophrenia, a sibling may experience such feelings as guilt, hurt, and anxiety. These experiences have been observed most commonly in younger, educated, and female siblings and the level of burden experienced by the caregiver may depend upon the severity of the patient's condition.

Family members may also find it difficult to recognize or acknowledge an illness that has been developing in their loved one, and this can sometimes lead to delays in seeking professional care. Other times, people with a mental disorder may hide their level of distress by being socially inclusive, which also hinders the initiation of professional intervention.

Studies suggest that psychoeducation can improve a family's ability to express emotions. This education can help to improve long-term functioning, which, in turn, can reduce the need for long-term caregiving. Home-based emergency interventions have also been found to reduce the burden placed on family members while improving interactions between family members and a loved one experiencing mental illness.

The behaviors exhibited by a person with a mental illness that has been shown to be of most concern to family members are:

- Impulsiveness
- Hyperactivity
- Insomnia
- Confusion
- Aggression
- Unpredictive behaviors

Not all people with a mental disability need a caregiver. But, family members are sometimes the ones who provide care for their loved ones who do. In such cases, the overall quality of life of the person experiencing mental illness will likely depend on the commitment of these family members.

Children of Parents with a Mental Illness

Children whose parents are affected by mental illness have been widely documented as the family members who take on the role of caregiver. This role could be limited to helping out or could involve extensive care. The effects this caregiving has on the child depends on multiple factors and can differ with each child, but their well-being may be impacted by this responsibility and attachments, such as love, care, and emotional nurturing may be at risk in such scenarios.

Siblings Whose Parents Have a Mental Illness

Researchers have also studied how a parent's mental disability affects an entire family. However, very little focus has been devoted to an examination of the relationships among siblings whose parent has been diagnosed with a mental disability. It has been noted that siblings often find solace and support in each other, especially during times when their parent's health is most at risk.

Siblings also may take on different roles in terms of caregiving. For example, the oldest sibling may look after the whole family if a parent is affected.

Mental illness is a common occurrence that affects people irrespective of gender, age, and socioeconomic status and its presence impacts entire families as well as individuals. Living with and caring for a person with a mental disability will have an impact on the well-being of not only the patient but also the family. Therefore, it is recommended that caregivers and affected family members work with mental-healthcare specialists to gain knowledge and understanding of the illness affecting their loved one as they provide familiar support.

References

1. Robinson, Elly; Rodgers, Bryan; and Butterworth, Peter. "Family Relationships and Mental Illness," Semantic Scholar, November 10, 2008.
2. "SHUT OUT: The Experience of People with Disabilities and their Families in Australia," Australian Government, Department of Social Services (DSS), September 19, 2016.
3. "Impact on Families," Neuroscience Research Australia (NeuRA), September 7, 2017.

Chapter 14 | HIV/AIDS and Mental Health

WHAT ARE HUMAN IMMUNODEFICIENCY VIRUS AND ACQUIRED IMMUNODEFICIENCY SYNDROME?

Human immunodeficiency virus or HIV is the virus that causes acquired immunodeficiency syndrome (AIDS). HIV attacks the immune system by destroying CD4 positive (CD4+) T cells, a type of white blood cell that is vital to fighting off infection. The destruction of these cells leaves people infected with HIV vulnerable to other infections, diseases, and other complications.

A person infected with HIV is diagnosed with AIDS when she or he has one or more opportunistic infections (which occurs when your immune system is damaged by HIV), such as pneumonia or tuberculosis, and has a dangerously low number of CD4+ T cells (less than 200 cells per cubic millimeter of blood).

People with HIV/AIDS are at a higher risk for mental-health disorders. If you are living with HIV, it is important for you to be aware that you have an increased risk for developing mood, anxiety, and cognitive disorders. For example, people living with HIV are twice as likely to have depression compared to those who are not infected with HIV. These conditions may be treatable. Many people with mental-health conditions recover completely.

Some forms of stress can contribute to mental-health problems for people living with HIV, including:

- Having trouble getting the services you need
- Experiencing a loss of social support, resulting in isolation

This chapter includes text excerpted from "HIV/AIDS and Mental Health," National Institute of Mental Health (NIMH), November 2016. Reviewed October 2019.

- Experiencing a loss of employment or worries about whether you will be able to perform your work as you did before
- Having to tell others you are HIV-positive
- Managing your HIV medicines
- Going through changes in your physical appearance or abilities due to HIV/AIDS
- Dealing with loss, including the loss of relationships or even death
- Facing the stigma and discrimination associated with HIV/AIDS

The HIV virus itself also can contribute to mental-health problems because it enters and resides in your brain. Some other opportunistic infections can also affect your nervous system and lead to changes in your behavior and functioning. Similarly, neuropsychological disorders, such as mild cognitive changes or more severe cognitive conditions, such as dementia, are associated with HIV disease.

You can better manage your overall health and well-being if you know how having HIV can affect your mental health and what resources are available to help you if you need them.

HUMAN IMMUNODEFICIENCY VIRUS-ASSOCIATED NEUROCOGNITIVE DISORDERS

Human immunodeficiency virus-associated neurocognitive disorders (HAND) represents the range of neurocognitive complications associated with HIV infection. Although there is currently no cure for HAND, combination antiretroviral therapy has been shown to be the only option in preventing or delaying the progression of HAND.

There are three major types of HAND:

- **Asymptomatic neurocognitive impairment (ANI)** is diagnosed if testing shows HIV-associated impairment in cognitive function, but everyday functioning is not affected.
- **Mild neurocognitive disorder (MND)** is diagnosed if testing shows HIV-associated impairment in cognitive function, and mild interference in everyday functioning.
- **HIV-associated dementia (HAD)** is diagnosed if testing shows marked impairment in cognitive function, especially

in the learning of information, information processing, and attention or concentration. This impairment significantly limits your ability to function day-to-day at work, home, and during social activities.

Although a significant proportion of people living with HIV are affected by a mild form of HAND, there has been significant progress in the treatment of HAND. Since the start of the epidemic, severe cases of HAND have been on the decline and the most severe form, HAD, is rare. The majority of people experience more subtle abnormalities in memory and cognition.

Experienced clinicians can diagnose HAND after carefully ruling out other possible causes of the symptoms. They may conduct a thorough neurological exam and history, neuropsychological testing, brain magnetic resonance imaging (MRI) scan, and sometimes lumbar puncture to evaluate the cerebrospinal fluid to obtain information about the nature and severity of HAND.

TREATMENTS AND THERAPIES

Research shows that HIV treatment should be initiated as soon as the infection is detected to achieve the best health outcomes. Once diagnosed, HIV infection is treated using a combination of medicines called "antiretroviral therapy" (ART). Adequate adherence to prescribed treatment regimens, such as taking the medications as prescribed by the healthcare provider, is critical to controlling the virus and to achieve complete viral suppression. Adequate adherence can be difficult but many strategies have been developed to assist individuals living with HIV/AIDS.

Starting antiretroviral therapy also can affect your mental health in different ways. Sometimes antiretroviral therapy can relieve your anxiety because knowing that you are taking care of yourself can give you a sense of security. However, coping with the reality of living with a chronic illness can be challenging. Depression is one of the most common mental-health conditions experienced by people living with HIV, just as it is in the general population. In addition, some antiretroviral medications may cause symptoms of depression, anxiety, and sleep disturbance, and may make some mental-health challenges worse.

For these reasons, it is important to talk to your healthcare provider about your mental health. A conversation about mental health should be part of your complete medical evaluation before starting antiretroviral medications. Continue to discuss your mental health with your healthcare team throughout treatment. Be open and honest with your provider about any changes in the way you are thinking, or how you are feeling about yourself and life in general. Also, discuss any alcohol or substance use with your provider so that she or he can help connect you to treatment if necessary.

In addition, tell your healthcare provider about any over-the-counter (OTC) or prescribed medications you may be taking, including any psychiatric medications, because some of these drugs may interact with antiretroviral medications.

Chapter 15 | **Attitudes toward Mental Illness and Stigma**

People's beliefs and attitudes toward mental illness set the stage for how they interact with, provide opportunities for, and help support a person with mental illness. People's beliefs and attitudes toward mental illness also frame how they experience and express their own emotional problems and psychological distress and whether they disclose these symptoms and seek care. About one in four U.S. adults (26.2%) age 18 and older, in any given year, has a mental disorder (e.g., mood disorder, anxiety disorder, impulse control disorder (ICD), or substance-abuse disorder, meaning that mental disorders are common and can affect anyone. Many adults with common chronic conditions, such as arthritis, cancer, diabetes, heart disease, and epilepsy experience concurrent depression and anxiety—further complicating self-management of these disorders and adversely affecting the quality of life (QOL).

Attitudes and beliefs about mental illness are shaped by personal knowledge about mental illness, knowing and interacting with someone living with mental illness, cultural stereotypes about mental illness, media stories, and familiarity with institutional practices and past restrictions (e.g., health insurance restrictions, employment restrictions; adoption restrictions). When such attitudes and beliefs are expressed positively, they can result in supportive and inclusive behaviors (e.g., willingness to date a person with mental illness or to hire a person with mental illness). When such attitudes and beliefs are expressed negatively, they may result in avoidance, exclusion from daily activities, and, in the worst case, exploitation and discrimination.

This chapter includes text excerpted from "Attitudes toward Mental Illness: Results from the Behavioral Risk Factor Surveillance System," Centers for Disease Control and Prevention (CDC), 2012. Reviewed October 2019.

Stigma has been described as "a cluster of negative attitudes and beliefs that motivate the general public to fear, reject, avoid, and discriminate against people with mental illnesses." When stigma leads to social exclusion or discrimination ("experienced" stigma), it results in unequal access to resources that all people need to function well: educational opportunities, employment, a supportive community, including friends and family, and access to quality healthcare. These types of disparities in education, employment, and access to care can have cumulative long-term negative consequences.

For example, a young adult with untreated mental illness who is unable to graduate from high school is less likely to find a good paying job that can support her or his basic needs, including access to healthcare. These disadvantages can cause a person to experience more negative outcomes. Being unemployed, living at or below the poverty line, being socially isolated, and living with other social disadvantages can further deflate self-esteem, compounding mental illness symptoms, and add to the burden of stigma. Sometimes stigma is simply "felt" in the absence of being discriminated against and results from internalizing perceived negative attitudes associated with a characteristic (e.g., age), a disorder (e.g., human immunodeficiency virus (HIV)/acquired immunodeficiency syndrome (AIDS)), a behavior (e.g., smoking), or other factor (e.g., place of birth).

Whether stigma is experienced as social exclusion or discrimination or felt as a pervasive and underlying sense of being different from others, it can be debilitating for people and poses a challenge for public health prevention efforts. Different opinions exist regarding the implications of different labels associated with describing mental illness (e.g., brain disease) and felt or experienced stigma. However, the prevailing view of health-related stigma is that it refers to perceived, enacted, or anticipated avoidance or social exclusion, and not to an individual blemish or mark. Different methods exist for measuring health-related stigma, and challenges and limitations associated with distinguishing between felt versus experienced stigma in attitudinal research have been described.

WHAT ARE THE CONSEQUENCES OF NEGATIVE ATTITUDES TOWARD MENTAL ILLNESS AND STIGMA?

Only about 20 percent of adults with a diagnosable mental disorder or with a self-reported mental-health condition saw a mental-health provider in the previous year. Embarrassment associated with accessing mental-health services is one of the many barriers that cause people to hide their symptoms and to prevent them from getting necessary treatment for their mental illness symptoms. Stigma poses a barrier for public health primary prevention efforts designed to minimize the onset of mental illness, as well as with secondary prevention efforts aimed at promoting early treatment to prevent worsening of symptoms over time.

Stigma can also interfere with self-management of mental disorders (tertiary prevention). Untreated symptoms can have grave consequences for people living with mental illness and negatively impact families affected by these disorders. For example, most people with serious and persistent mental illness (mental disorders that interfere with some area of social functioning) are unemployed and live below the poverty line, and many face major barriers to obtaining decent, affordable housing. These individuals may need a number of additional social supports (e.g., job training, peer-support networks) to live successfully in the community, but such supports may not be available. Other individuals with depression and anxiety might avoid disclosing their symptoms and instead adopt unhealthy behaviors to help them cope with their distress (e.g., smoking, excessive alcohol use, binge-eating). These behaviors can increase their risk for developing chronic diseases, worsening their overall health over time. Some studies have found an increased risk of death at younger ages for people with mental illness.

Attitudes toward mental illness can also influence how policymakers allocate public resources to mental-health services, pose challenges for staff retention in mental-health settings, result in poorer quality of medical care administered to people with mental illness, and create fundraising challenges for organizations who serve people with mental illness and their families. State-level factors such as unemployment levels and access to mental-health services, and the presence or absence of other state resources may affect public attitudes and merit study.

WHY IS IT IMPORTANT TO TRACK ATTITUDES TOWARD MENTAL ILLNESS?

People's attitudes and beliefs predict their behavior. People's beliefs and attitudes about mental illness might predict whether they disclose their symptoms and seek treatment and support. Knowledge and beliefs that can aid in the recognition, management, or prevention of mental-health disorders are defined as mental-health literacy. Tracking attitudes toward mental illness can serve as an indicator of the public's mental-health literacy. For example, in a 1996 study, 54 percent of the U.S. public attributed major depression to neurobiological causes, and this increased to 67 percent in 2006. Similarly, a larger percentage of people endorsed the benefits of treatment by a physician for people with major depression in 2006 (91%) than in 1996 (78%). However, improvements in neurobiological understanding of mental illness were unrelated to negative attitudes and, in some cases, increased the odds of negative attitudes (e.g., need for social distance, perceived dangerousness). In another study of U.S. adults, only about one fourth agreed that people are caring and sympathetic to people with mental illness. When asked about how much it would be worth to avoid mental illness compared to general medical illnesses, the public was less willing to pay to avoid mental-health treatment than they were to pay to avoid physical health treatment. These studies provide important snapshots of attitudes toward mental illness across the country; however, studies that examine attitudes in-depth such as distinguishing between attitudes relative to perceived or experienced stigma, studies that link attitudes to actual behavior, or studies that track attitudes toward mental illness at the state level do not occur routinely. These limited, cross-sectional studies tell us little about how attitudes shift in relation to historical events (e.g., media over sensationalization of the rare violence associated with a person with mental illness), how attitudes shift over time in the same people, and how these attitudes differ within a state relative to characteristics of the state such as the average unemployment rate or per capita expenditures on state mental-health agencies.

Chapter 16 | Media Portrayal of Mental Illness

Today, more people than ever use media technology, such as smartphones, laptops, and televisions as they go about their daily lives. This means that, unless a person majored in psychology, social work, or attended medical school, their impression of a person with a mental disability has been deeply informed by depictions found in newspapers, films, television shows, and on social media. Yet media depictions of mental illness are inaccurate more often than not.

Studies suggest that media is one of the primary sources of information that the American public rely on to inform their opinions about mental illnesses, such as bipolar disorder, schizophrenia, and depression, and the people who live day in and day out with these disorders. Yet most media portrayals of mental illness are cynical, stigmatizing, and simply incorrect. These inaccurate portrayals also may discourage people from seeking the services of a mental-health professional; since media representation can lead users to believe that mental-health treatment is only meant for people with an extreme behavioral or psychiatric disorder.

COMMON MISCONCEPTIONS OF PERSON WITH A MENTAL ILLNESS

Some common misconceptions about mental illness that are influenced by media depictions are listed below:

- A person with a mental disability is immoral or aggressive.
- A person with a mental illness looks different than other people.
- A person with a mental illness is irrational.
- All people with mental illness behave in a similarly erratic way.

- Psychiatric hospitals cause more harm than good.
- Mental illness is a lifelong problem that can neither be treated nor cured.

MEDIA AND THE STIGMA OF MENTAL ILLNESS

Distinguishing fact from fiction is especially important when stigma is associated with such misconceptions. While it is true that many members of the U.S. population are affected by mental illness, most recover from or are able to manage their symptoms and go on to live full and meaningful lives. But, the social stigma associated with mental illness also can result in people with a mental disorder experiencing widespread and harmful prejudice.

Almost 9 out of 10 people with a mental-health diagnosis report that stigma associated with their condition has had a negative impact on their lives. The extent of this harm is reflected in the reality that a person with a mental disability is less likely to:

- Have a job
- Find a long-time or life partner
- Maintain a stable home life
- Be included in social activities

This stigma also may worsen a person's condition by affecting their treatment progress or delaying their actually seeking treatment.

Studies indicate that the best way to move past such media-driven negative stereotyping of people with a mental disorder is to open direct lines of communication with people who have experienced mental-health symptoms. Encouraging such social interactions can be accomplished through awareness programs that shift the public's attitude toward mental illness and thereby reduce stigma.

PORTRAYAL OF MENTAL ILLNESS IN MEDIA, FILMS, AND BOOKS

A majority of therapists in films and books are portrayed as exhibiting more mental-health symptoms than their patients. These composite characters often are depicted as being agitated, irrational, and arrogant. Naturally, some therapists will face problems of their own from time to time, just as many of us will, but this depiction is distorted.

Although it is rare, some movies and books do portray mental illness authentically, however, and showcase the actual ways in which therapists and psychiatric healthcare providers operate. This is especially true when a particular mental-health condition, such as depression and schizophrenia, is showcased.

MEDIA AND SUBSTANCE-USE DISORDER

Media also has a strong influence on how members of the general population view drugs and substance-use disorder (SUD). The drug-related stories in myriad newspapers, films, magazines, books, and on television often present people as requiring these substances in order to function. These people are often portrayed as someone who became instantly addicted to a harmful substance and whose addiction led to increasingly violent behaviors that ultimate led to social and economic destruction. As with inaccurate depictions of mental illness, this stereotyping of people with a SUD may lead many to believe that only people who are highly dependent on substances need to seek treatment that could help them enjoy a healthier and more satisfying quality of life.

Media not only negatively brands people with a SUD in ways that are harmful and inaccurate, but also tends to convey information related to addiction from a negative, disapproving, and moralizing viewpoint. And portrayals such as these have a high chance of increasing the likelihood that people who are dealing with a SUD will experience negative consequences.

MEDIA AND SUICIDE

Research indicates that certain media portrayals of suicide also may trigger suicidal thoughts in consumers who are vulnerable to such influences and thereby increase the rate of suicide. Research further suggests that modifying the media's approach to its depictions of mental illness may decrease suicide rates. The positive effect that the media has on people is known as the "Papageno effect," and the negative effect is known as the "Werther effect." Based on studies of the effect media has on people, various guidelines are now in place to reduce the risk of suicide traceable to media influence.

Some guidelines that the media can follow to reduce suicide risk follow:

- Avoid generalizations
- Avoid phrases that sensationalize mental illness
- Consider the effects the news will have on people, including the family, friends, and loved ones of people with a mental disorder
- Include information on how viewers can find immediate help if they or someone they know is experiencing suicidal thoughts or feelings when reporting about suicide
- Avoid presenting suicide as a front-page headline
- Avoid mentioning personal information, such as the full name and photograph of someone who has committed or attempted to commit suicide, in media stories
- Emphasize the negative outcomes of intentional self-harm, which may prevent future suicides

REPORTING MENTAL ILLNESS

A well-researched media report about mental illness can help members of the general population understand the disorder more accurately. Media outlets are encouraged to present their content in an accurate, responsible, and well-balanced manner:

- Offer an empathetic view of people living with a mental illness to decrease the likelihood that media consumers will become desensitized to the needs of people living with a mental disability.
- Give hope by sharing the success stories of people who have lived with and recovered from a mental illness.
- Encourage people who have a mental illness to seek immediate help.
- Provide precise and clear information regarding any type of mental illness that is reported.

Mass media and its tremendous reach have the power to influence the public in both positive or harmful ways and the manner in which mental illness is portrayed can lead to stigmatization and the perpetuation of harmful myths about mental illness or can inform others of the details of how professional psychiatric intervention can alleviate symptoms and improve overall quality of life. Reporting stories about mental illness in a balanced and accurate manner will help others understand the complexities and treatment of mental illness while reducing the risk of suicide among mentally ill people.

References

1. "Media and Mental Health," National Center for Biotechnology Information (NCBI), June 2018.
2. "Stigma and Discrimination," Mental Health Foundation, February 25, 2011.
3. Tartakovsky, Margarita. "The Media and Mental Illness: The Good, the Bad and the Ridiculous," Psych Central, December 15, 2011.
4. "How Mental Illness Is Misrepresented in the Media," U.S. News & World Report, April 16, 2015.
5. "Stigmatization of People with Addictive Disorders," Dianova International, July 5, 2018.

Chapter 17 | Should You Disclose Your Mental Illness to Your Employer?

If you have a mental illness, are age 18 through 64, receive Social Security disability benefits, and are considering work, this information is for you! Social Security's Ticket to Work program provides free support to help you find and keep a job and become financially independent, to the greatest extent possible. For information, contact the Ticket to Work Help Line at 866-968-7842 (V) or 866-833-2967 (Toll-free TTY), Monday through Friday from 8 a.m. to 8 p.m. Eastern time (ET). Ask an agent to send you a list of service providers. You can also search for providers online using the "Find Help (choosework.ssa.gov/findhelp/)" tool. When you find a provider who meets your needs and agrees to work with you, it will help you develop a plan to reach your employment goal. Your provider will probably also talk with you about disability disclosure.

To tell or not to tell—that is the question. According to the National Alliance on Mental Illness (NAMI), nearly one in five people will experience a diagnosable mental-health condition, such as depression, anxiety, bipolar disorder, and schizophrenia or have trouble dealing with some form of significant distress. Depression is one of the most widespread forms of mental illness and 70 percent of people with depression are in the workforce. Despite the prevalence, the fear of stigma and discrimination on the job remains high. It is no surprise that many adults struggle with the issue of disability disclosure.

This chapter includes text excerpted from "Should You Disclose Your Mental Illness to Your Employer?" U.S. Social Security Administration (SSA), May 31, 2016. Reviewed October 2019.

On one hand, disclosing your diagnosis may relieve you of the feeling that you need to hide your condition and, in fact, may equip you with resources to better perform your job. As a person with a disability, you are entitled to protections under the Americans with Disabilities Act (ADA) and can request job accommodations, such as modified duties, job site, and work hours. Finally, disclosing your disability may create an opportunity for your employer to educate your supervisors and coworkers about your symptoms and dispel myths about mental illness.

On the other hand, workplace disclosure carries some risks. Although confidentially is guaranteed, you may determine that the possibility of your personal information getting into the wrong hands is too great to take the chance. You may worry that if you share your diagnosis with your employer or potential employer that your chances of being promoted or hired will decrease, and that supervisors and coworkers may have negative reactions and may, mistakenly, see you as less capable.

It is definitely a tough call. Any decision regarding disclosure of your mental-health condition is your decision. If you decide to disclose, you may choose to be open with everyone or to tell only your immediate supervisor or specific coworkers. Keep in mind, there is no specific time frame required to reveal a mental illness to an employer. Take all the time needed to determine if disclosing your condition to your employer is the right choice for you. Understand, though, if you need reasonable accommodations, your employer is not required to provide them until you disclose your condition or how it affects you.

Work can change your life. Weigh the pros and cons of disclosure and decide what is right for you.

Chapter 18 | Youth Transitioning with Mental Disability

Starting a job can be difficult for any young person. If you happen to have a hidden disability, such as a mental-health impairment, a new workplace can be overwhelming. If you have ever felt this way, you are not alone. According to the National Institute of Mental Health (NIMH), the leading cause of disability in the United States for ages 15 to 44 is major depressive disorder (MDD) (and this is only one type of mental-health impairment). Along with questions about the job itself, you may have questions about when and how to disclose your disability. You may wonder if it is appropriate to ask for modifications in your new work setting. This chapter provides guidance to assist you with a successful transition into the workforce by answering questions regarding disclosure, accommodations, and resources.

THE AMERICANS WITH DISABILITIES ACT AND YOUTH WITH MENTAL-HEALTH IMPAIRMENTS

The Americans with Disabilities Act (ADA) was signed into law in 1990. It is a federal civil rights law protecting people with disabilities from discrimination, including youth with mental-health impairments. The law has different sections called "Titles." Each Title addresses discrimination in different settings. The section regarding discrimination against people with disabilities in the workplace is called "Title I." This section prohibits discrimination in all aspects

This chapter includes text excerpted from "Entering the World of Work: What Youth with Mental Health Needs Should Know about Accommodations," U.S. Department of Labor (DOL), April 11, 2007. Reviewed October 2019.

of employment, including recruitment, preemployment screening, hiring, compensation, benefits, training, layoffs, termination, and promotions and requires that most employers provide reasonable accommodations for qualified job applicants and employees with known disabilities. A reasonable accommodation is any change in the work environment or in the way things are usually done which enables a person with a disability to perform the essential functions of the job.

The term "disability" is defined as:

- A physical or mental impairment that substantially limits one or more major life activities
- A record of a physical or mental impairment that substantially limits one or more major life activities, or
- Being regarded as having a physical or mental impairment that substantially limits one or more major life activities

Sometimes it can be difficult to know whether Title I of the ADA applies to you. If you are a person with a mental-health disability, Title I applies to you when you are "qualified" for a job. Being qualified means you have the required skill, experience, education, and other job-related requirements for the position. You are qualified if you can perform the important or essential job tasks of the position, even if you need a reasonable accommodation to do so. It is important to note that, if you are applying to work at a small business, the ADA only applies to employers with 15 or more workers.

COMMON ON-THE-JOB CONCERNS FOR YOUTH WITH MENTAL-HEALTH DISABILITIES

As you start your new job, it is important to know that many youth with mental-health disabilities share similar experiences. Common challenges include:

- Maintaining regular attendance
- Dealing with the change of starting a new job
- Nervousness about interacting with others
- Understanding how to manage time
- Organizing information
- Handling stress and emotions
- Maintaining focus

This list does not include all experiences youth with mental-health disabilities may face. Job tasks you find challenging because of your disability may be adjusted or modified through requesting accommodations from your employer. However, before you ask for an accommodation, you need to know a little bit about disclosing your disability.

DISCLOSING YOUR MENTAL-HEALTH DISABILITY

Disclosing your disability in an employment setting is ultimately a personal decision and can change depending upon the situation and the need for accommodation.

You only need to disclose your disability if you want to ask for an accommodation to complete the application process or to do job-related tasks. Disclosure is necessary to receive a reasonable accommodation because most employers are legally required to provide accommodations for a job applicant or worker with a known disability.

If you do not need accommodation, disclosing your disability is completely your decision. You should do what you think is best. Always trust yourself regarding disclosure. When and if you choose to tell your employer you have a disability, you should do it in a way that is comfortable for you. Asking people close to you for their opinions on how to disclose your disability may be helpful, but ultimately you should do what you feel is right. If you choose to disclose, focus your discussion on what you can do, not what you cannot do.

REQUESTING AN ACCOMMODATION

Many employers are aware of accommodations for people with physical disabilities, but may not know how to accommodate people with invisible disabilities. Unlike in high school, it is your responsibility to ask for an accommodation. You need to be aware of your individual needs and abilities and be able to communicate them to your employer.

People with disabilities can request an accommodation at any time during the application process or while employed. To request an accommodation, you have to inform your employer of the need for an adjustment or change at work for a reason related to your disability.

Table 18.1. Common Challenges and Possible Accommodations

Challenge	Possible Accommodations
Maintaining consistent attendance	• Flexible leave to attend counseling • Making up time missed • Schedule a later start time
Dealing with change	• Maintaining open lines of communication with supervisor • Scheduling regular meetings with supervisor to discuss work-related issues
Interacting with others	• Providing a mentor, a team leader or a buddy to facilitate social and work-related interactions • Participating in team activities
Managing time	• An electronic calendar marked with meetings and deadlines • Use E-mail as a time management tool • Daily or weekly performance goals • A partner or a mentor to help with time management
Organizing information	• Assistance in prioritizing tasks • A written to-do list, which can be reviewed on a regular basis • Dividing large assignments into smaller tasks • A personal data assistant or other electronic organizer
Handling stress and emotions	• Short breaks to walk around the block • Praise and positive reinforcement • Permission to call or instant message a support person
Maintaining concentration	• A quiet location • Space enclosures • Wearing a headset or ear sets and listening to music or "white noise"

There are no keywords you must use in order to make the request, and neither the ADA nor the phrase "reasonable accommodation" has to be mentioned. Do not be afraid to ask your employer for work-related accommodation if it will help you perform your job better.

SOME COMMON TYPES OF REASONABLE ACCOMMODATIONS

Below are some common challenges and possible accommodations you might ask your employer to consider. If you decide to disclose your disability and ask your employer for an accommodation, it is a good idea to have already considered what type of accommodation you need to better perform your job. This list may help you think about possible solutions.

Chapter 19 | Working with a Mental-Health Condition

Millions of Americans living with mental-health conditions lead happy, successful lives. People with very serious mental-health and substance-abuse problems might have trouble with basic needs, like finding a place to live, a job, or healthcare.

HOW CAN I FIND A JOB?

Many people with mental-health conditions can and do work. Finding a job you enjoy can help improve your mental health and give you a sense of purpose. Studies show that most adults with serious or severe mental-health conditions want to work and about 6 out of 10 can succeed with the right kind of support. More than 1 in every 4 women who work have a disability of some type (a physical disability or a mental-health condition).

Women whose mental-health conditions have affected their ability to accomplish daily tasks may have more trouble finding a job, especially if they have been out of the workforce for a long time. If you do not have a full-time job right now, you may want to try a part-time job or volunteering before committing to full-time work. You can also take an online test, called a "skills assessment" or an "interest assessment," which can help you learn more about the types of work you might enjoy.

Check with the mental-health agency where you receive mental-health services. Your state may offer several different ways to find employment, including:

- **Vocational rehabilitation (rehab) services.** Rehabilitation services help a person with a serious mental-health

This chapter includes text excerpted from "Working with a Mental Health Condition," Office on Women's Health (OWH), U.S. Department of Health and Human Services (HHS), August 28, 2018.

condition or disability find and keep a job. Different states and communities have different requirements for who is eligible to get vocational rehab services.

- **Supported employment.** This type of program helps people with serious mental illnesses (SMI) get jobs in the community and be successful in the workplace.
- **Clubhouses.** Clubhouses are settings that allow people with serious mental-health conditions to live and work together, providing services and support to one another.
- **Local public employment office.** The U.S. Department of Labor (DOL) operates employment offices in all 50 states. You can find job counselors and information about opportunities available in your area. Visit the DOL's service locator to find an office near you.

IF I CANNOT WORK, WHAT DO I DO ABOUT MONEY?

If you are unable to work because of a mental-health condition or any other disability, there are some options for financial support. These include disability insurance and disability payments through Social Security.

- **Disability insurance.** Some people purchase disability insurance policies, either on their own or through their employer, before a disability happens. If you have been paying each month into a disability insurance policy and now you are disabled and cannot work, you may be able to receive payments.
- **Social Security Income (SSI).** SSI is cash assistance for people who have little to no income. The amount of cash you receive from SSI depends on your other income and living arrangements. The standard amount is about $700 per month for an individual, but your payment may be more or less, depending on where you live and what other help you may get. To find out whether you qualify for SSI benefits, visit the U.S. Social Security Administration (SSA) website (www.ssa.gov/ssi) or call the SSA at 800-772-1213.
- **Social Security Disability Insurance (SSDI).** SSDI provides monthly income to people who become disabled by a

physical or mental-health condition before retirement age. More than one in three people who receive SSDI get it because of a mental-health condition.

If you are a member of the military, you can get your Social Security application processed faster.

HOW DO I PAY FOR TREATMENT?

Most health plans cover preventive services, like depression screening for adults and behavioral assessments for children, at no additional cost. Most health-insurance plans must cover treatment for mental-health and substance-use problems in the same ways medical or surgical problems are covered.

- If you have insurance, contact your insurance provider to find out what is included in your plan.
- If you have Medicaid, your plan will provide some mental-health services and may offer services to help with substance-use disorders (SUDs).
- If you have Medicare, your plan may help cover mental-health services, including hospital stays, visits to a therapist, and medicines you may need.

If you do not have insurance, see whether you are eligible for free or low-cost health insurance (including Medicaid or the Children's Health Insurance Plan (CHIP)) at HealthCare.gov.

SHOULD I TELL PEOPLE I WORK WITH THAT I HAVE A MENTAL-HEALTH CONDITION?

There is no law that requires you to share personal-health information, including mental-health conditions, with anyone you work with. Telling others about your mental-health condition can affect your job in the future. If you want to tell someone you work with about your mental-health illness, think about your reasons carefully. It might help to make a list of the good and bad outcomes of telling your manager or someone in human resources.

Your employer must make reasonable accommodations if they know about your mental-health condition, but employers do not have to accommodate disabilities that they do not know about. This may help you decide whether you tell your employer about your mental-health condition.

Learn more reasons to tell or not tell your employer about a mental-health condition from the U.S. Equal Employment Opportunity Commission (EEOC) and the National Alliance on Mental Illness (NAMI).

WHAT LAWS PROTECT PEOPLE WITH DISABILITIES

Many federal laws protect the rights of people with disabilities, including mental-health conditions. The main law is the Americans with Disabilities Act (ADA). It mostly protects people from discrimination at work and in public places and programs.

Under the ADA, you are protected if:

- Your mental-health condition (if left untreated) interferes with your ability to get things done at home or at work
- You can perform the essential functions of a job you have or hope to get, with or without reasonable accommodations (such as a flexible work schedule)

Other laws that protect people with disabilities include:

- **The Fair Housing Act.** This law makes it illegal to deny housing to a renter or buyer because of a disability. Owners must also make reasonable accommodations to people with disabilities.
- **The Individuals with Disabilities Education Act (IDEA).** This law requires that free public education be made available to children and youth with disabilities. It also requires that education be designed to meet their unique educational needs.
- **The Rehabilitation Act of 1973.** This law is very broad and requires that all federal programs, activities, and employment be accessible to people with disabilities. It served as the foundation for the ADA and helps people with disabilities become employed and independent.

HOW DOES THE AMERICANS WITH DISABILITIES ACT PROTECT ME AT WORK?

The Americans with Disabilities Act (ADA) protects you from discrimination based on disability, including harassment related to disability. For example, you cannot be fired just because you take medicine for a mental-health condition. However, an employer can fire you for poor performance. It is better to ask for reasonable accommodations before a disability causes problems with job performance. Under the ADA:

Your employer must make reasonable accommodations if they know about your mental-health condition. Your employer is allowed to ask for documentation from a healthcare professional about your condition. The documentation does not need to be detailed.

- Employers do not have to accommodate disabilities that they do not know about. This may help you decide whether you tell your employer about your mental-health condition.
- If your employer knows about your disability and you are having a difficult time doing your job, your employer is allowed to ask whether you need reasonable accommodations.
- An employer cannot legally ask questions about your medical or psychiatric history during an interview.
- An employer is allowed to ask you questions that help the employer decide whether you can perform the essential duties of a job. An employer may ask you about your ability to meet the physical requirements for jobs involving physical labor, your ability to get along with people, or your ability to finish tasks on time and to come to work every day.

WHAT IS AN EXAMPLE OF REASONABLE ACCOMMODATION AT WORK FOR SOMEONE WITH A MENTAL-HEALTH CONDITION?

Examples of reasonable accommodations for people with mental-health conditions may include:

- Providing self-paced workloads and flexible hours
- Adjusting your job responsibilities
- Allowing leave (paid or unpaid) if you are hospitalized or temporarily unable to work
- Assigning a flexible, supportive, and understanding supervisor
- Changing your work hours to allow you to attend psychiatrist or therapist appointments

- Providing more support or supervision, such as writing to-do lists and checking in more often with your supervisor

An employer does not have to provide these specific accommodations, but these types of accommodations are often considered reasonable for some jobs.

WHAT DO I DO IF I HAVE BEEN DISCRIMINATED AGAINST BECAUSE OF MY MENTAL-HEALTH CONDITION?

If you have experienced employment discrimination because of your mental-health condition, you can file an administrative charge or complaint with the EEOC or a state or local antidiscrimination agency. You can also file a lawsuit in the court, but only after filing an administrative charge.

The Fair Housing Act bars discrimination in rental housing for people with disabilities. This means that property owners or managers cannot refuse to rent to you because of a disability, including mental-health conditions. If you believe you have been discriminated against, you can file a housing complaint online through the Fair Housing Act.

WHAT STEPS CAN I TAKE TO PROTECT MY MENTAL HEALTH?

During stressful times like job and housing transitions, you can try the following tips to stay mentally healthy:

- **Take your medicines.** If you take medicines for a mental-health condition, do not stop taking them without first talking with your doctor or nurse.
- **Have a plan.** Learn about the things that help you feel well and about the things that cause you to feel stressed. Develop a plan so that you can identify warning signs that your mental or physical health might be slipping and an action plan for getting the support you need to stay well.
- **Get enough sleep.** Lack of sleep can affect your mental and physical health. It can also make it more difficult to cope with mental-health conditions.
- **Reach out to your support network.** Tell your friends and family if you are going through something such as a job or housing transition. Ask for help if you need it.

- **Be physically healthy.** Getting active, quitting smoking, limiting alcohol, and eating the right amount of healthy foods from across the food groups help your body and mind feel better.
- **Get professional help.** Keep your appointments with a mental-health professional, such as a therapist, counselor, or social worker. This person can help notice signs of mental-health conditions getting worse.

Chapter 20 | **Link between Poverty and Mental Illness**

The prevalence of poverty in the United States is an important public health issue. In 2015, approximately 43 million Americans lived in poverty. Although the U.S. Census Bureau uses "a set of dollar value thresholds that vary by family size and composition to determine who is in poverty," poverty may be defined in a number of different ways, particularly by socioeconomic status (SES).

SERIOUS MENTAL ILLNESS AMONG ADULTS BELOW THE POVERTY LINE

The challenges that adults with mental illness face are made more difficult if they are living in poverty. For example, adults with mental illness who are living in poverty may face higher healthcare costs, decreased productivity, and poor general health. According to the National Survey of Drug Use and Health (NSDUH), an estimated 9.8 million adults aged 18 or older in the United States had a serious mental illness (SMI), including 2.5 million adults living below the poverty line. SMI is defined in NSDUH as adults who in the past year have had a diagnosable mental, behavioral, or emotional disorder (excluding developmental and substance use disorders (SUDs)) of sufficient duration to meet diagnostic criteria and has resulted in serious functional impairment substantially interferes with major life activities. Adults aged 26 or older living below the poverty line were more likely to experience SMI than those living at and above

This chapter contains text excerpted from the following sources: Text in this chapter begins with excerpts from "Poverty," Office of Disease Prevention and Health Promotion (ODPHP), U.S. Department of Health and Human Services (HHS), September 29, 2018; Text under the heading "Serious Mental Illness among Adults below the Poverty Line" is excerpted from "Serious Mental Illness among Adults below the Poverty Line," Substance Abuse and Mental Health Services Administration (SAMHSA), November 15, 2016. Reviewed October 2019.

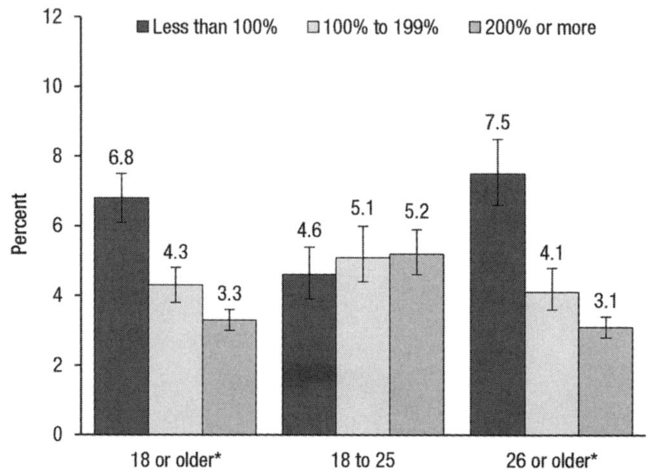

Figure 20.1. Serious Mental Illness among Adults Aged 18 and Older by Poverty Status: 2015 National Survey on Drug Use and Health (NSDUH)

Note: Error bars visually represent the variability or uncertainty in the percentages.

the poverty line (7.5% versus. 4.1 and 3.1%, respectively). In contrast, the percentage of young adults with SMI was similar in each of the levels of poverty.

The relationship between mental illness and poverty is complicated. Poverty may intensify the experience of mental illness. Poverty may also increase the likelihood of the onset of mental illness. At the same time, experiencing a mental illness may also increase the chances of living below the poverty line.

Part 3 | **Recovery, Rehabilitation, and Caregiving**

Chapter 21 | Recovery Model and Treatment of Mental Illness

RECOVERY IS POSSIBLE

Most people with mental-health challenges can get better. Treatment and recovery are ongoing processes that happen over time. The first step is getting help.

What Is Recovery?

Recovery from mental disorders and/or substance-abuse disorders is a process of change through which individuals:

- Improve their health and wellness
- Live a self-directed life
- Strive to achieve their full potential

Four Dimensions of Recovery

Four major dimensions support a life in recovery:

1. **Health.** Make informed, healthy choices that support physical and emotional well-being.
2. **Home.** Have a stable and safe place to live.
3. **Purpose.** Engage in meaningful daily activities, such as a job or school, volunteering, caring for your family, or being

This chapter contains text excerpted from the following sources: Text under the heading "Recovery Is Possible" is excerpted from "Recovery Is Possible," MentalHealth.gov, U.S. Department of Health and Human Services (HHS), March 14, 2019; Text under the heading "Recovery and Recovery Support" is excerpted from "Recovery and Recovery Support," Substance Abuse and Mental Health Services Administration (SAMHSA), May 17, 2019.

creative. Work for independence, income, and resources to participate in society.

4. **Community.** Build relationships and social networks that provide support.

Develop a Recovery Plan

If you are struggling with a mental-health challenge, you may want to develop a written recovery plan.

Recovery plans:

- Enable you to identify goals for achieving wellness
- Specify what you can do to reach those goals
- Include daily activities as well as longer-term goals
- Track any changes in your mental-health challenge
- Identify triggers or other stressful events that can make you feel worse, and help you learn how to manage them
- Get information about Partners for Recovery (PFR), which provides technical resources to those who deliver services for mental-health and substance-abuse conditions.

RECOVERY AND RECOVERY SUPPORT

Recovery-oriented care and recovery support systems help people with mental and substance-use disorders (SUDs) manage their conditions successfully.

There are four major dimensions that support recovery:

1. **Health**—overcoming or managing one's disease(s) or symptoms and making informed, healthy choices that support physical and emotional well-being
2. **Home**—having a stable and safe place to live
3. **Purpose**—conducting meaningful daily activities and having the independence, income, and resources to participate in society
4. **Community**—having relationships and social networks that provide support, friendship, love, and hope

Hope, the belief that these challenges and conditions can be overcome, is the foundation of recovery. The process of recovery is highly personal and occurs via many pathways. Recovery is characterized by continual growth and improvement in one's health and wellness that may involve setbacks. Because setbacks are a natural part of life, resilience becomes a key component of recovery.

The process of recovery is supported through relationships and social networks. This often involves family members who become the champions of their loved one's recovery. Families of people in recovery may experience adversities that lead to increased family stress, guilt, shame, anger, fear, anxiety, loss, grief, and isolation. The concept of resilience in recovery is also vital for family members who need access to intentional supports that promote their health and well-being. The support of peers and friends is also crucial in engaging and supporting individuals in recovery.

Recovery services and supports must be flexible. What may work for adults may be very different for youth or older adults. For example, the nature of social supports, peer mentors, and recovery coaching for adolescents is different than for adults and older adults. Supporting recovery requires that mental health and addiction services:

- Be responsive and respectful to the health beliefs, practices, and cultural and linguistic needs of diverse people and groups
- Actively address diversity in the delivery of services
- Seek to reduce health disparities in access and outcomes

The Substance Abuse and Mental Health Services Administration (SAMHSA) established recovery support systems to promote partnering with people in recovery from mental and SUDs and their family members to guide the behavioral-health system and promote individual, program, and system-level approaches that foster health and resilience (including helping individuals with behavioral health needs be well, manage symptoms, and achieve and maintain abstinence); increase housing to support recovery; reduce barriers to employment, education, and other life goals; and secure necessary social supports in their chosen community.

The SAMHSA demonstrates that behavioral health is essential to health, prevention works, treatment is effective, and people recover from mental and/or SUDs.

Chapter 22 | Recovery after an Initial Schizophrenia Episode (RAISE) Project: Questions and Answers

WHAT IS RECOVERY AFTER AN INITIAL SCHIZOPHRENIA EPISODE?

In 2008, the National Institute of Mental Health (NIMH) launched the Recovery After an Initial Schizophrenia Episode (RAISE) Project. RAISE is a large-scale research initiative that began with two studies examining different aspects of coordinated specialty care (CSC) treatments for people who were experiencing first-episode psychosis. One study focused on whether or not the treatment worked better than care typically available in community settings. The other project studied the best way for clinics to start using the treatment program. The goal of RAISE was, and is, to help decrease the likelihood of future episodes of psychosis, reduce long-term disability, and help people to get their lives back on track so they can pursue their goals. The two RAISE studies are no longer enrolling participants. Current efforts are focused on sharing information learned from the original studies and looking for additional ways to improve the lives of people experiencing first-episode psychosis. RAISE researchers are exploring new areas, such as identifying ways of decreasing the duration of untreated psychosis.

This chapter includes text excerpted from "RAISE Questions and Answers," National Institute of Mental Health (NIMH), October 7, 2015. Reviewed October 2019.

WHY IS RECOVERY AFTER AN INITIAL SCHIZOPHRENIA EPISODE IMPORTANT?

The RAISE project was designed to study the best ways to intervene after a person begins to experience psychotic symptoms, such as hallucinations, delusions, or disorganized speech. The goal is to change the downward spiral that can result from untreated psychosis, and help return people to a path toward productive, independent lives. Preventing negative events like dropping out of school, losing the ability to work, and losing contact with friends and family also has the potential to reduce indirect costs to society. The two RAISE projects studied the CSC treatment model in a large number of real-world clinics, so results are relevant to many community treatment settings throughout the United States.

WHAT IS THE RECOVERY AFTER AN INITIAL SCHIZOPHRENIA EPISODE EARLY TREATMENT PROGRAM?

The RAISE Early Treatment Program (RAISE-ETP) was one of two research projects that made up the NIMH RAISE initiative. RAISE-ETP was a clinical trial that enrolled more than 400 people at 34 clinics across the United States. It compared NAVIGATE, a CSC treatment program for first-episode psychosis, to care typically found in community clinics. The RAISE-ETP study team designed the NAVIGATE treatment program, and put it into practice at "real-world" clinics across the country, training existing clinical staff to provide NAVIGATE services. The goal of the clinical trial was to determine whether people in the NAVIGATE program had better outcomes than people at clinics that provided typical care. John M. Kane, M.D., vice president (VP) for behavioral health services of the North Shore-Long Island Jewish (LIJ) Health System and chairman of psychiatry at the Zucker Hillside Hospital led the RAISE-ETP study.

WHAT DID WE LEARN FROM THE RECOVERY AFTER AN INITIAL SCHIZOPHRENIA EPISODE EARLY TREATMENT PROGRAM STUDY?

The RAISE-ETP findings show that over two years, clients at the NAVIGATE clinics stayed in treatment longer; experienced greater improvement in their symptoms, interpersonal relationships, and quality of life (QOL); and were more involved in work or school compared to clients at the typical-care sites. NAVIGATE clients who had a shorter duration of untreated psychosis (DUP) when they started the study showed even greater improvements than those with longer DUP. RAISE-ETP researchers will continue to study factors that might influence clients' outcomes. The study showed that coordinated specialty care for first-episode psychosis can be used in a variety of U.S. community mental-health clinics. For state health administrators, the tools and manuals that supported the NAVIGATE treatment program are available online.

WHAT IS THE RECOVERY AFTER AN INITIAL SCHIZOPHRENIA EPISODE IMPLEMENTATION AND EVALUATION STUDY?

The RAISE Implementation and Evaluation Study (RAISE-IES) was one of two research projects that made up NIMH's RAISE initiative. RAISE-IES explored how to implement a specially designed CSC treatment called the "Connection Program." The researchers created two specialty care clinics for treating first-episode psychosis, one in New York and one in Maryland. The project examined the clinical and administrative aspects of establishing such specialty care clinics and developed tools and materials that others may use to start their own CSC programs. The study also looked at factors that affected clients' and family members' satisfaction with treatment, as well as clients' outcomes after participating in the Connection Program. Dr. Lisa Dixon, M.D., professor of psychiatry at Columbia University in New York and the director of the Center for Practice Innovations (CPI) at the New York State Psychiatric Institute (NYSPI) led RAISE-IES.

WHAT DID WE LEARN FROM RECOVERY AFTER AN INITIAL SCHIZOPHRENIA EPISODE IMPLEMENTATION AND EVALUATION STUDY?

The RAISE-IES produced important information that helps us understand how to make a CSC treatment program work for both clinics and clients. For state administrators, or those interested in starting their own CSC program, the RAISE-IES developed tools and resources to help achieve this goal. For example, in addition to treatment manuals and program guides, RAISE-IES developed practical strategies for monitoring treatment fidelity. In other words, RAISE-IES developed ways of checking to see if the clinic actually provided the treatment program as it was intended to be delivered. Knowing how to do this is important since fidelity data help clinical administrators maintain high-quality programs. Fidelity data also help clients and families know if they are getting the CSC services they expect and the data help those paying for CSC services, such as insurers, know if clients are getting the services they are paying for. To address the issue of how to sustain a program over the long term, RAISE-IES showed it was possible to partner with state mental-health authorities in order to pay for CSC services and to expand the number of clinics available.

The RAISE-IES study compared clients' functioning at initial contact to outcomes two years later, showing promising results for individuals participating in the CSC program. Clients' symptoms improved over time as did their work, educational and social lives. Finally, researchers showed that the CSC treatment model was appealing. Clients participated and stayed in the CSC program because they felt they were treated with warmth and respect and because they received effective services.

Chapter 23 | Peer Support and Recovery

WHAT IS PEER SUPPORT?

Peer support encompasses a range of activities and interactions between people who have shared similar experiences of being diagnosed with mental-health conditions. This mutuality—often called "peerness"—between a peer worker and person using services promotes connection and inspires hope.

Peer support offers a level of acceptance, understanding, and validation not found in many other professional relationships. "I am an expert at not being an expert, and that takes a lot of expertise," said one (anonymous) peer worker, highlighting the supportive rather than directive nature of the peer relationship. By sharing their own lived experience and practical guidance, peer workers help people to develop their own goals, create strategies for self-empowerment, and take concrete steps toward building fulfilling, self-determined lives for themselves.

WHAT DO PEER SUPPORT SPECIALISTS DO?

Support the Recovery of Individuals

Peer workers offer encouragement, practical assistance, guidance, and understanding to support recovery. Peer support workers walk alongside people in recovery, offering individualized supports and demonstrating that recovery is possible. They share their own lived experience of moving from hopelessness to hope. They share tools that can complement or replace clinical supports by providing strategies for self-empowerment and achieving a self-determined life.

This chapter contains text excerpted from the following sources: Text beginning with the heading "What Is Peer Support?" is excerpted from "Value of Peers Infographics: Peer Support," Substance Abuse and Mental Health Services Administration (SAMHSA), November 26, 2017; Text under the heading "How Does Peer Support Help" is excerpted from "Value of Peers, 2017," Substance Abuse and Mental Health Services Administration (SAMHSA), November 17, 2017.

They support people in recovery to connect with their own inner strength, motivation, and desire to move forward in life, even when experiencing challenges. Peer workers offer different types of support, including:

- **Emotional** (empathy and camaraderie)
- **Informational** (connections to information and referrals to community resources that support health and wellness)
- **Instrumental** (concrete supports such as housing or employment)
- **Affiliational support** (connections to community supports, activities, and events)

Improve Mental-Health Systems

Peer support is valuable not only for the person receiving services but also for behavioral health professionals and the systems in which they work. Peer workers educate their colleagues and advance the field by sharing their perspectives and experience in order to increase understanding of how practices and policies may be improved to promote wellness and resiliency. This is particularly important in mental-health systems, where historical oppression, violence, and discrimination present significant barriers to recovery for many people. Peer workers play vital roles in moving behavioral health professionals and systems towards recovery orientation.

HOW DOES PEER SUPPORT HELP

The role of a peer support worker complements but does not duplicate or replace the roles of therapists, case managers, and other members of a treatment team. Peer support workers bring their own personal knowledge of what it is like to live and thrive with mental-health conditions and substance-use disorders (SUDs). They support people's progress towards recovery and self-determined lives by sharing vital experiential information and real examples of the power of recovery. The sense of mutuality created through thoughtful sharing of experience is influential in modeling recovery and offering hope.

Chapter 24 | Guiding Principles of Recovery

RECOVERY EMERGES FROM HOPE

The belief that recovery is real provides the essential and motivating message of a better future—that people can and do overcome the internal and external challenges, barriers, and obstacles that confront them. Hope is internalized and can be fostered by peers, families, providers, allies, and others. Hope is the catalyst for the recovery process.

RECOVERY IS PERSON-DRIVEN

Self-determination and self-direction are the foundations for recovery as individuals define their own life goals and design their unique path(s) towards those goals. Individuals optimize their autonomy and independence to the greatest extent possible by leading, controlling, and exercising choice over the services and supports that assist their recovery and resilience. In so doing, they are empowered and provided the resources to make informed decisions, initiate recovery, build on their strengths, and gain or regain control over their lives.

RECOVERY OCCURS VIA MANY PATHWAYS

Individuals are unique with distinct needs, strengths, preferences, goals, culture, and backgrounds—including trauma experience—that affect and determine their pathway(s) to recovery. Recovery is built on the multiple capacities, strengths, talents, coping abilities, resources, and inherent value of each individual. Recovery pathways

This chapter includes text excerpted from "SAMHSA's Working Definition of Recovery," Substance Abuse and Mental Health Services Administration (SAMHSA), April 15, 2010. Reviewed October 2019.

are highly personalized. They may include professional clinical treatment; use of medications; support from families and in schools; faith-based approaches; peer support; and other approaches. Recovery is nonlinear, characterized by continual growth and improved functioning that may involve setbacks. Because setbacks are a natural, though not inevitable, part of the recovery process, it is essential to foster resilience for all individuals and families. Abstinence from the use of alcohol, illicit drugs, and nonprescribed medications is the goal for those with addictions. The use of tobacco and nonprescribed or illicit drugs is not safe for anyone. In some cases, recovery pathways can be enabled by creating a supportive environment. This is especially true for children, who may not have the legal or developmental capacity to set their own course.

RECOVERY IS HOLISTIC

Recovery encompasses an individual's whole life, including mind, body, spirit, and community. This includes addressing: self-care practices, family, housing, employment, transportation, education, clinical treatment for mental disorders and substance use disorders, services and supports, primary healthcare, dental care, complementary and alternative services, faith, spirituality, creativity, social networks, and community participation. The array of services and supports available should be integrated and coordinated.

RECOVERY IS SUPPORTED BY PEERS AND ALLIES

Mutual support and mutual aid groups, including the sharing of experiential knowledge and skills, as well as social learning, play an invaluable role in recovery. Peers encourage and engage other peers and provide each other with a vital sense of belonging, supportive relationships, valued roles, and community. Through helping others and giving back to the community, one helps one's self. Peer-operated supports and services provide important resources to assist people along their journeys of recovery and wellness. Professionals can also play an important role in the recovery process by providing clinical treatment and other services that support individuals in their chosen recovery paths. While peers and allies play an important role for many in recovery, their role for children and youth may be slightly different. Peer supports for families are very important for children with behavioral health problems and can also play a supportive role for youth in recovery.

RECOVERY IS SUPPORTED THROUGH RELATIONSHIP AND SOCIAL NETWORKS

An important factor in the recovery process is the presence and involvement of people who believe in the person's ability to recover; who offer hope, support, and encouragement; and who also suggest strategies and resources for change. Family members, peers, providers, faith groups, community members, and other allies form vital support networks. Through these relationships, people leave unhealthy and/or unfulfilling life roles behind and engage in new roles (e.g., partner, caregiver, friend, student, employee) that lead to a greater sense of belonging, personhood, empowerment, autonomy, social inclusion, and community participation.

RECOVERY IS CULTURALLY BASED AND INFLUENCED

Culture and cultural background in all of its diverse representations—including values, traditions, and beliefs—are keys in determining a person's journey and unique pathway to recovery. Services should be culturally grounded, attuned, sensitive, congruent, and competent, as well as personalized to meet each individual's unique needs.

RECOVERY IS SUPPORTED BY ADDRESSING TRAUMA

The experience of trauma (such as physical or sexual abuse, domestic violence, war, disaster, and others) is often a precursor to or associated with alcohol and drug use, mental-health problems, and related issues. Services and supports should be trauma-informed to foster safety (physical and emotional) and trust, as well as promote choice, empowerment, and collaboration.

RECOVERY INVOLVES INDIVIDUAL, FAMILY, AND COMMUNITY STRENGTHS AND RESPONSIBILITY

Individuals, families, and communities have strengths and resources that serve as a foundation for recovery. In addition, individuals have a personal responsibility for their own self-care and journeys of recovery. Individuals should be supported in speaking for themselves. Families and significant others have responsibilities to support their loved ones, especially for children and youth in recovery. Communities have responsibilities to provide opportunities and resources to address discrimination and to foster social inclusion and recovery. Individuals in recovery also have a social responsibility and should have the ability to join with peers to speak collectively about their strengths, needs, wants, desires, and aspirations.

RECOVERY IS BASED ON RESPECT

Community, systems, and societal acceptance and appreciation for people affected by mental-health and substance use problems—including protecting their rights and eliminating discrimination—are crucial in achieving recovery. There is a need to acknowledge that taking steps towards recovery may require great courage. Self-acceptance, developing a positive and meaningful sense of identity, and regaining belief in one's self are particularly important.

Chapter 25 | **Healthy Lifestyle to Support Recovery**

Section 25.1 | Physical Activity and Mental Health

This section contains text excerpted from the following sources: Text in this section begins with excerpts from "Why Physical Activity Is Important," girlshealth.gov, Office on Women's Health (OWH), March 27, 2015. Reviewed October 2019; Text beginning with the heading "How Does Physical Activity Affect Your Mental Health?" is excerpted from "Steps to Support Good Mental Health," Office on Women's Health (OWH), U.S. Department of Health and Human Services (HHS), August 28, 2018.

You may wonder if being physically active is really worth the time and effort. Well, lots of girls think so! They know being active is a great way to have fun and hang out with friends. And fitness can do some pretty amazing things for your mind and body.

WHAT BEING ACTIVE DOES FOR YOUR MENTAL HEALTH?

Did you know being physically active can affect how good you feel? It also can affect how well you do your tasks, and even how pleasant you are to be around. That is partly because physical activity gets your brain to make "feel-good" chemicals called "endorphins." Regular physical activity may help you by:

- Reducing stress
- Improving sleep
- Boosting your energy
- Reducing symptoms of anxiety and depression
- Increasing your self-esteem
- Making you feel proud for taking good care of yourself
- Improving how well you do at school

WHAT BEING ACTIVE DOES FOR YOUR BODY?

Being physically active is great for your muscles, heart, and lungs. It may even help with the premenstrual syndrome (PMS) symptoms. Some other possible benefits of activity include:

- **Building strong bones.** Your body creates the most bone when you are a kid and a teen.
- **Promoting a healthy weight.** Obesity is a serious problem among kids in the United States. It can lead to problems with your sleep, knees, heart, emotions, and more, but exercise can help.

- **Helping avoid diabetes.** A lot more young people are getting diabetes than ever before. Regular physical activity can help prevent one type of diabetes.
- **Building healthy habits.** If you get used to being active now, you will more likely keep it up when you are older.
- **Fighting cancer.** Research shows that exercise may help protect against certain kinds of cancer, including breast cancer.
- **Helping prevent high blood pressure.** The number of kids with high blood pressure is growing. High blood pressure makes your heart and arteries work extra hard to pump blood. It also puts you at risk for things such as kidney and eye disease.

Are you worried that exercise will bulk you up? Exercising would not give you big, bulging muscles. It takes a very intense weightlifting program to get a body-builder look. Exercise and other forms of physical activity can help if you need to lose weight or want to stay a healthy weight.

HOW DOES PHYSICAL ACTIVITY AFFECT YOUR MENTAL HEALTH?

Physical activity can help your mental health in several ways:

- **Aerobic exercise can boost your mood.** Your body makes certain chemicals, called "endorphins," during and after your workout. Endorphins relieve stress and make you feel calmer.
- **Getting physical activity during the day can make it easier to sleep at night.** Creating a routine can help you stay motivated and build a habit of getting regular physical activity.
- **Physical activity may help with depression and anxiety symptoms.** Studies show that regular aerobic exercise boosts your mood and lowers anxiety and depression.
- **Physical activity may help slow or stop weight gain,** which is a common side effect of some medicines used to treat mental-health conditions.

Regular physical activity can benefit your health over the long term. Getting active every day (at least 30 minutes a day of moderate-intensity aerobic activity, such as brisk walking) helps maintain your health. All Americans should also do strengthening exercises at least two days a week to build and maintain muscles. Your doctor or nurse may recommend exercise in addition to taking medicine and getting counseling for mental-health conditions.

HOW DOES YOUR PHYSICAL HEALTH AFFECT YOUR MENTAL HEALTH?

People who are not physically healthy may have trouble staying mentally healthy. People living with chronic (long term) health problems such as diabetes and heart disease are often more likely to have higher stress levels, depression, and anxiety. Researchers are not sure which problems happen first, but many people have a chronic disease and a mental-health condition. Having a chronic disease does not always mean you will have a mental-health condition, but if you are struggling with both, know that you are not alone. Support groups and healthcare professionals can help. Healthy habits, such as eating healthy and getting exercise, that help improve many chronic diseases may also help improve mental-health conditions.

Section 25.2 | Eating Well and Mental Health

This section contains text excerpted from the following sources: Text in this section begins with excerpts from "Importance of Good Nutrition," President's Council on Sports, Fitness & Nutrition (PCSFN), U.S. Department of Health and Human Services (HHS), January 26, 2017; Text under the heading "How Does What You Eat and Drink Affect Your Mental Health?" is excerpted from "Steps to Support Good Mental Health," Office on Women's Health (OWH), U.S. Department of Health and Human Services (HHS), August 28, 2018.

Your food choices each day affect your health—how you feel today, tomorrow, and in the future.

Good nutrition is an important part of leading a healthy lifestyle. Combined with physical activity, your diet can help you to reach and maintain a healthy weight, reduce your risk of chronic diseases (such as heart disease and cancer), and promote your overall health.

THE IMPACT OF NUTRITION ON YOUR HEALTH

Unhealthy eating habits have contributed to the obesity epidemic in the United States: about one-third of U.S. adults (33.8%) are obese and approximately 17 percent (or 12.5 million) of children and adolescents aged 2 to 19 years are obese. Even for people at a healthy weight, a poor diet is associated with major health risks that can cause illness and even death. These include heart disease, hypertension (high blood pressure), type 2 diabetes, osteoporosis, and certain types of cancer. By making smart food choices, you can help protect yourself from these health problems.

The risk factors for adult chronic diseases, such as hypertension and type 2 diabetes, are increasingly seen in younger ages, often a result of unhealthy eating habits and increased weight gain. Dietary habits established in childhood often carry into adulthood, so teaching children how to eat healthy at a young age will help them stay healthy throughout their life.

The link between good nutrition and healthy weight reduced chronic disease risk, and overall health is too important to ignore. By taking steps to eat healthily, you will be on your way to getting the nutrients your body needs to stay healthy, active, and strong. As with physical activity, making small changes in your diet can go a long way.

HOW DOES WHAT YOU EAT AND DRINK AFFECT YOUR MENTAL HEALTH?

The foods you eat and what you drink can have a direct effect on your energy levels and mood. Researchers think that eating healthier foods can have a positive effect on your mood.

- Getting the right balance of nutrients, including enough fiber and water, can help your mood stay stable. Sugary, processed foods increase your blood sugar and then make you feel tired and irritable when your blood sugar levels drop.
- Some vitamins and minerals may help with the symptoms of depression. Experts are researching how a lack of some nutrients is linked to depression in new mothers.
- These include selenium, omega-3 fatty acids, folate, vitamin B_{12}, calcium, iron, and zinc.

- Drinking too much alcohol can lead to mental and physical health challenges.
- Drinks with caffeine can make it harder for you to sleep, which can make some mental-health conditions worse. Also, drinking caffeine regularly and then suddenly stopping can cause caffeine withdrawal, which can make you irritable and give you headaches. Do not have drinks with caffeine within five hours of going to sleep.

Eating nutritious foods may not cure a mental-health condition, but eating healthy is a good way to start feeling better. Ask your doctor or nurse for more information about the right foods to eat to help keep your mind and body healthy.

Section 25.3 | Sleep and Mental Health

This section includes text excerpted from documents published by two public domain sources. Text under the headings marked 1 are excerpted from "Sleep and Your Health," Office on Women's Health (OWH), U.S. Department of Health and Human Services (HHS), March 14, 2019; Text under the headings marked 2 are excerpted from "Get Enough Sleep," Office of Disease Prevention and Health Promotion (ODPHP), U.S. Department of Health and Human Services (HHS), July 18, 2018.

SLEEP AND YOUR HEALTH[1]

Sleep affects your mental and physical health. Getting good sleep helps boost your mind and mood and can help prevent health problems. Women are more likely than men to have insomnia and other sleep problems. Changing hormones during the menstrual cycle, pregnancy, and menopause can affect how well a woman sleeps. But, there are steps you can take to get the rest you need.

HOW MUCH SLEEP DO CHILDREN NEED?[2]

Kids need even more sleep than adults.

- Teens need 8 to 10 hours of sleep each night

- School-aged children need 9 to 12 hours of sleep each night
- Preschoolers need to sleep between 10 and 13 hours a day (including naps)
- Toddlers need to sleep between 11 and 14 hours a day (including naps)
- Babies need to sleep between 12 and 16 hours a day (including naps)

HOW MUCH SLEEP DO ADULTS NEED?[2]

Most adults need seven to eight hours of good quality sleep on a regular schedule each night. Make changes to your routine if you cannot find enough time to sleep.

Getting enough sleep is not only about total hours of sleep. It is also important to get good quality sleep on a regular schedule so you feel rested when you wake up.

If you often have trouble sleeping—or if you often still feel tired after sleeping—talk with your doctor.

WHY IS GETTING ENOUGH SLEEP IMPORTANT?[2]

Getting enough sleep has many benefits. It can help you:

- Get sick less often
- Stay at a healthy weight
- Lower your risk for serious health problems, such as diabetes and heart disease
- Reduce stress and improve your mood
- Think more clearly and do better in school and at work
- Get along better with people
- Make good decisions and avoid injuries—for example, sleepy drivers cause thousands of car accidents every year

DOES IT MATTER WHEN YOU SLEEP?[2]

Yes. Your body sets your "biological clock" according to the pattern of daylight where you live. This helps you naturally get sleepy at night and stay alert during the day.

If you have to work at night and sleep during the day, you may have trouble getting enough sleep. It can also be hard to sleep when you travel to a different time zone.

Get sleep tips to help you:

- Work the night shift
- Deal with jet lag (trouble sleeping in a new time zone)

WHY CANNOT YOU FALL ASLEEP?[2]

Many things can make it harder for you to sleep, including:

- Stress or anxiety
- Pain
- Certain health conditions, such as heartburn or asthma
- Some medicines
- Caffeine (usually from coffee, tea, and soda).
- Alcohol and other drugs
- Untreated sleep disorders, such as sleep apnea or insomnia

If you are having trouble sleeping, try making changes to your routine to get the sleep you need. You may want to:

- Change what you do during the day—for example, get your physical activity in the morning instead of at night
- Create a comfortable sleep environment—and make sure your bedroom is dark and quiet
- Set a bedtime routine—and go to bed at the same time every night

HOW CAN YOU TELL IF YOU HAVE A SLEEP DISORDER?[2]

Sleep disorders can cause many different problems. Keep in mind that it is normal to have trouble sleeping every now and then. People with sleep disorders generally experience these problems on a regular basis.

Common signs of sleep disorders include:

- Trouble falling or staying asleep
- Still feeling tired after a good night's sleep
- Sleepiness during the day that makes it difficult to do everyday activities, such as driving a car or concentrating at work
- Frequent loud snoring
- Pauses in breathing or gasping while sleeping

- Itchy feelings in your legs or arms at night that feel better when you move or massage the area
- Trouble moving your arms and legs when you wake up

If you have any of these signs, talk to a doctor or nurse. You may need to be tested or treated for a sleep disorder.

HOW DOES SLEEP AFFECT YOUR MENTAL HEALTH?[1]

Your mind and body are healthier when you sleep well. Your body needs time every day to rest and heal. Some sleep disorders, such as insomnia, sleep apnea, and restless leg syndrome (RLS), make it harder to fall asleep or stay asleep. This can lead to daytime sleepiness and make it more difficult to stay in good mental health.

Having a sleep problem can also trigger a mental-health condition or make current mental-health conditions worse. Also, mental-health conditions or treatments can sometimes cause sleep problems.

Section 25.4 | Smoking Cessation and Recovery Outcome

This section includes text excerpted from "What We Know: Tobacco Use and Quitting among Individuals with Behavioral Health Conditions," Centers for Disease Control and Prevention (CDC), January 14, 2019.

TOBACCO USE AND QUITTING AMONG INDIVIDUALS WITH BEHAVIORAL HEALTH CONDITIONS

Nearly 25 percent of adults in the United States have a mental-health or substance-use disorder (SUD) (i.e., behavioral health condition), and these adults consume almost 40 percent of all cigarettes smoked by adults in the United States.

People with behavioral health conditions die about five years earlier than people without such conditions, more than 50 percent from tobacco-attributable diseases.

The first step in addressing tobacco use among individuals with behavioral health conditions is understanding the available evidence.

People with behavioral health conditions:

1. **Are more likely to smoke.** Individuals with a behavioral health condition are more likely to smoke than people without such a condition, and smoking rates are even higher among individuals with serious mental-health disorders and addictions.
2. **Smoke more.** Individuals with behavioral health conditions smoke more cigarettes than people who smoke and do not have these conditions.
3. **Want to quit smoking.** Many individuals with behavioral health conditions want to quit smoking but may face extra challenges in successfully quitting and may benefit from extra help.
4 **Die prematurely.** Individuals with serious mental-health disorders who smoke die almost 15 years earlier than individuals without these disorders who do not smoke.
5. **Die from a smoking-related illness.** People with behavioral health conditions account for over 200,000, or nearly half, of tobacco-related deaths each year. The most common causes of death among people with behavioral health conditions are heart disease, cancer, and lung disease, all of which can be caused by smoking.

Smoking among people with behavioral health conditions:

1. **Exacerbates symptoms of behavioral health conditions.** Smoking is associated with worse symptoms and outcomes among people with behavioral health conditions, including greater depressive symptoms, greater likelihood of psychiatric hospitalization, increased suicidal behavior, and drug and alcohol-use relapse.
2. **Reduces the effectiveness of some medications.** Smoking can interact and interfere with psychiatric medications, often resulting in the need for higher medication doses to achieve the same therapeutic benefit.

The Case for Tobacco Cessation Treatment

Behavioral health treatment settings have permitted tobacco use among clients, in part because of misperceptions that smoking could alleviate the symptoms of mental-health conditions and that cessation could interfere with treatment. However, research has shown that smoking can worsen symptoms and behavioral health outcomes, and quitting can improve mental-health and substance-use disorder treatment outcomes.

Quitting tobacco:

1. **Supports behavioral health treatment.** Growing evidence indicates that quitting smoking has positive effects on and is associated with improvements in mental health. Quitting smoking does not interfere with behavioral health treatment and does not worsen or impede recovery from substance-use disorders (SUDs).
2. **Could improve mental health.** Quitting smoking is associated with a decrease in depression, anxiety, and stress, and can increase the quality of life (QOL).
3. **Could make relapse less likely.** Quitting smoking is associated with an increase in long-term abstinence from alcohol and other drugs and a reduction in substance-use disorder relapse.
4. **Has immediate physical health benefits.** Quitting smoking dramatically reduces the risk of heart disease, stroke, and cancer. For example, the risk for a heart attack drops sharply just one year after quitting.

Chapter 26 | Supported Employment for Serious Mental Illness

Over two-thirds of individuals with serious mental illness (SMI) want to work and indicate that finding appropriate employment opportunities is a top priority. In addition to providing income, the opportunity to work facilitates social inclusion and influences many aspects of health status. For people with disabilities, employment can serve to increase self-esteem, social integration, and participation in community activities. Employment is viewed as a primary treatment goal for people with a psychiatric disability. For these reasons, the employment of individuals with SMI is being measured as part of the Healthy People 2020 objectives, a set of scientific objectives for improving the health of Americans, which are measured over a 10-year period.

Despite the widespread recognition that employment is a crucial component of recovery, prevalence estimates from the National Survey on Drug Use and Health (NSDUH) indicate that the proportion of individuals with SMI (i.e., those surveyed who live in households and met criteria for a diagnosable mental illness with substantial impairment) who were employed fell from 56.0 percent in 2008 to 48.5 percent in 2013. This decline is in contrast to substantial improvement in the overall U.S. employment rate during the same period. Employment rates are found to be even lower among individuals receiving public mental-health services, ranging from 17.9 percent to 39.0 percent depending on the definition of the sample.

This chapter includes text excerpted from "Availability of Supported Employment in Specialty Mental Health Treatment Facilities and Facility Characteristics: 2014," Substance Abuse and Mental Health Services Administration (SAMHSA), June 15, 2017.

Many people with a psychiatric disability want to work and could be successful in achieving competitive employment with the help of an evidence-based supported employment service known as "Individual Placement and Support" (hereafter referred to as supported employment).

Supported employment is an important intervention that can enable people with SMI to succeed in finding and maintaining jobs. Supported employment services differ from traditional vocational rehabilitation services. Supported employment focuses on achieving outcomes by matching individuals to jobs best suited for their skills, strengths, interests, and capacities, and by providing continuous support during employment. Vocational rehabilitation focuses on career counseling, job-seeking skills, training, and assistance navigating job markets. More specifically, supported employment uses eight guiding principles, which distinguishes it from other vocational support programs:

- Every person who wants to work is eligible.
- Competitive jobs are the goal.
- Supported employment services are integrated with mental-health services.
- Personalized benefits counseling is provided (to address concerns about the potential loss of health benefits and disability payments).
- The job search starts soon after a person expresses interest in working (there is no requirement of readiness other than interest).
- Employment specialists build relationships with employers (individuals receive more than employment leads).
- Individualized job supports are time unlimited (before and during employment).
- Individual preferences are honored (this effectively focuses the job search on positions that use an individual's strengths and skills and that are aligned with her or his interests).

Along with psychotherapy, medication, family support, and education, and case management supported employment can play a key role in a successful recovery. Moreover, supported employment in itself can be the main motivating factor for which an individual with SMI seeks treatment; individuals may not be ready to admit that they have an illness, but if they are struggling with employment they may accept help from programs that offer supported employment. However, despite the strong evidence base supporting this type of intervention, recent surveys of state mental-health authorities indicate that only about two percent of adults with SMI have access to supported employment.

Specialty mental-health treatment facilities provide an ideal setting for individuals with SMI to receive supported employment services. Using data from the most recent national survey, the goal of this report is to describe the number and characteristics of specialty mental-health treatment facilities that offered supported employment in the United States.

Chapter 27 | Importance of Psychological Resilience in Recovery

A great deal of literature exists in both the mental and substance-use disorder (SUD) fields about building, enhancing, and activating resilience in persons at risk for and with mental and/or SUDs. Many of the resilience studies that have been conducted have focused on children, adolescents, and young adults—populations that are greatly influenced by family, peers, and social environments revolving largely around the individual's school, community, and neighborhood.

Resilience, as a concept and construct, is the context-specific ability to respond to stress, anxiety, trauma, crisis, or disaster. Resilience develops over time and is the culmination of multiple internal and external factors. For those who developmental and/or SUDs, the influence of both internal development and external environments converge to either promote or restrict the development of personal resilience. The work of enhancing resilience for persons with mental and/or substance-use problems has its greatest impact during the formative stages to prevent more severe conditions and to promote health. Additionally, although more research is needed to fully examine the possible effects, resilience is also critical in the recovery stage where life skills and other supports can be accessed to manage future stress. It is the interaction of risk and protective

This chapter contains text excerpted from the following sources: Text in this chapter begins with excerpts from "Resilience Annotated Bibliography—SAMHSA's Partners for Recovery Initiative, March 2013," Substance Abuse and Mental Health Services Administration (SAMHSA), March 2013. Reviewed October 2019; Text beginning with the heading "What Is Individual Resilience?" is excerpted from "Individual Resilience," Office of the Assistant Secretary for Preparedness and Response (ASPR), U.S. Department of Health and Human Services (HHS), January 29, 2018.

factors that plays a central role in the development, enhancement, and activation of resilience.

Protective factors, which may exist or be developed in individuals, families, communities, and environments, reduce the impact of risk factors and enhance one's ability to "bounce back." Protective factors can be defined as specific circumstances, experiences, and resources that ameliorate a person's reaction to a situation that, in ordinary circumstances, might lead to maladaptive behaviors and outcomes. Protective factors may include:

- **Individual factors**, such as development of a desirable personal identity; a feeling of power and control over one's life; a feeling of self-worth; a sense of social justice; a sense of cohesion with others; good self-regulation skills; close relationships with competent adults; connections to prosocial organizations; tolerance for delayed gratification; a sense of humor; development of good coping and problem-solving skills; an ability to see and set long-term goals; and a positive outlook for the future.
- **Family factors**, such as consistent, appropriate parental involvement, discipline, and supervision; good parenting skills; trusting relationships; a safe environment; well-defined and appropriate family roles and responsibilities; opportunities to learn to deal appropriately with criticism, rejection, and silence; prosocial values and ethics; and good goal-setting and decision-making skills exhibited by parents.
- **Community factors**, such as participation in school, work, and the community that create an environment in which an individual has opportunities to develop and practice social and cognitive skills, develop a sense of belonging, contribute to the work of the community, develop a social network of peers, and learn to handle challenges and practice prosocial behavioral skills and self-efficacy.

Risk factors come in many different forms, but at their core, they are attitudes, beliefs, or environmental circumstances that put an individual in jeopardy of developing a mental and/or SUD. Depending on the source, risk factors may include:

- **Individual temperament characteristics** related to locus of control (external versus internal), poor self-control, negative emotionality, a need for immediate gratification, and even physical activity level
- **Family-related risk factors**, which may include parental and sibling drug use, poor child-rearing and socialization practices, ineffective parental supervision of the child, ineffective parental discipline skills, negative parent-child relationships, family conflict, marital discord, domestic violence, abuse and neglect, family disorganization, and family social isolation
- **Community/environmental risk factors** or the social determinants of health, e.g., limited resources, low socioeconomic status, and communities that lack the knowledge, skills, and programming necessary to reach out to those in need of assistance

Although the impact of a single protective or risk factor may have little effect on the individual, a combination of risk factors, for example, can create multilevel stress events that can overwhelm individuals who do not have a well-developed resilience to stress and lack the coping, decision-making, and problem-solving skills necessary to bounce back.

Understanding the role of risk and protective factors resonate with current health reforms that focus on prevention and community wellness, which in turn influence the social determinants of health. The risk and protective factors involved in building, enhancing, and activating resilience in persons with or at risk for behavioral health conditions form the foundations of the social determinants of health.

WHAT IS INDIVIDUAL RESILIENCE?

Individual resilience involves behaviors, thoughts, and actions that promote personal well-being and mental health. People can develop the ability to withstand, adapt to, and recover from stress and adversity—and maintain or return to a state of mental-health well-being—by using effective coping strategies. It is called "individual resilience."

A disaster can impair resilience due to stress, traumatic exposure, distressing psychological reactions, and disrupted social networks. Feelings of grief, sadness, and a range of other emotions are common after traumatic events. Resilient individuals, however, are able to work through the emotions and effects of stress and painful events and rebuild their lives.

WHAT CONTRIBUTES TO INDIVIDUAL RESILIENCE

People develop resilience by learning better skills and strategies for managing stress and better ways of thinking about life's challenges. To be resilient one must tap into personal strengths and the support of family, friends, neighbors, and/or faith communities.

WHAT ARE THE CHARACTERISTICS THAT SUPPORT INDIVIDUAL RESILIENCE?

Age, gender, health, biology, education level, cultural beliefs and traditions, and economic resources can play important roles in psychological resilience. The following characteristics also contribute to individual resilience:

- **Social support and close relationships with family and friends.** People who have close social support and strong connections with family and friends are able to get help during tough times and also enjoy their relationships during everyday life.
- **The ability to manage strong feelings and impulses.** People who are able to manage strong emotions are less likely to get overwhelmed, frustrated, or aggressive. People who are able to manage feelings can still feel sadness or loss, but they are also able to find healthy ways to cope and heal.
- **Good problem-solving skills.** People problem-solve daily. Thinking, planning, and solving problems in an organized way are important skills. Problem-solving skills contribute to feelings of independence and self-competence.
- **Feeling in control.** After the chaos of a disaster, it can be useful to engage in activities that help people regain a sense of control. This will help support the healing and recovery process.

- **Asking for help and seeking resources.** Resourceful people will get needed help more quickly if they know how to ask questions, are creative in their thinking about situations, are good problem solvers and communicators, and have a good social network to reach out to.
- **Seeing yourself as resilient.** After a disaster, many people may feel helpless and powerless, especially when there has been vast damage to the community. Being able to see yourself as resilient, rather than as helpless or as a victim, can help build psychological resilience.
- **Coping with stress in healthy ways.** People get feelings of pleasure and self-worth from doing things well. Strategies that use positive and meaningful ways to cope are better than those which can be harmful, such as drinking too much or smoking.
- **Helping others and finding positive meaning in life.** Positive emotions like gratitude, joy, kindness, love, and contentment can come from helping others. Acts of generosity can add meaning and purpose to your life, even in the face of tragedy.

Resilient individuals are able to:

- Care for themselves and others day-to-day and during emergency situations
- Actively support their neighborhoods, workplaces, and communities to recover after a disaster
- Be confident and hopeful about overcoming present and future difficulties
- Get needed resources more effectively and quickly
- Be physically and mentally healthier and have overall lower recovery expenses and service needs
- Miss fewer days of work
- Maintain stable family and social connections
- Reestablish routines more quickly, which helps children and adults alike

WAYS TO STRENGTHEN RESILIENCE

You can build your resilience by taking care of your health, managing stress, and being an active participant in the life of your community. For example, try to:

- Develop coping skills and practice stress management activities, such as yoga, exercise, and meditation.
- Eat healthy and exercise
- Get plenty of sleep
- Maintain social connections to people and groups that are meaningful for you
- Volunteer in your community
- Get training in first aid, cardiopulmonary resuscitation (CPR), community emergency response team (CERT), and psychological first aid
- Create evacuation and family reunification plans
- Make a disaster kit and stock supplies to shelter in place for up to three days
- Find things that bring you pleasure and enjoyment, such as reading a book or watching a movie, writing in a journal, or engaging in an art activity

DOES INDIVIDUAL RESILIENCE HELP BUILD COMMUNITY RESILIENCE?

Yes! Individual resilience is important to community resilience in that healthy people make for a healthier community. Healthy communities are better able to manage and recover from disasters and other emergencies.

Chapter 28 | Rehabilitation Medicine

WHAT IS REHABILITATION MEDICINE?

Rehabilitation medicine describes efforts to improve function and minimize impairment related to activities that have been hampered by disease, injuries, or developmental disorders.

Injuries, illnesses, or conditions that may cause or contribute to disability can include stroke, traumatic brain injury (TBI), spinal cord injury (SCI), musculoskeletal injuries, pain, a number of intellectual and developmental disorders, such as cerebral palsy (CP), fragile X syndrome (FXS), and autism spectrum disorders (ASDs), and other conditions and injuries.

The primary effects of many such conditions are physical—perhaps mobility or sensory problems. But individuals facing them can also experience intellectual, behavioral, and communication difficulties. They might have problems with making decisions, paying attention, or speaking. These can also require rehabilitation medical care.

Rehabilitation medicine differs from drug and alcohol rehabilitation, which aims to help a person control or eliminate her or his substance use, and from the rehabilitation that is commonly referred to within the context of the criminal justice system.

WHY MIGHT SOMEONE NEED REHABILITATION MEDICINE?

There are many reasons why a person may need care related to rehabilitation medicine. For example:

- Injuries and trauma, such as:
  - Burns

This chapter includes text excerpted from "Rehabilitation Medicine: Topic Information," *Eunice Kennedy Shriver* National Institute of Child Health and Human Development (NICHD), December 1, 2016. Reviewed October 2019.

    - Limb loss or amputation
    - Fractures, including multiple fractures to the long bones in the limbs and fractures of the hip, spine, or skull
    - Traumatic brain injury or concussion (mild TBI)
    - Spinal cord injury
    - Loss of sight or hearing
- Diseases and conditions that can cause loss of mobility function, such as:
    - Muscular dystrophy (MD)
    - Spina bifida (SB)
    - Cerebral palsy
    - Arthritis
    - Scoliosis or curvature of the spine
    - Damage to muscles, ligaments, tendons, or cartilage
    - Knee arthroplasty/replacement
    - Hip replacement
    - Stroke
    - Multiple sclerosis (MS)
    - Parkinson disease (PD) and related degenerative disorders
- Surgery or prolonged treatment for other diseases or illnesses that can cause loss of function, such as:
    - Chronic pain/neuropathy
    - Severe infection
    - Diabetes
    - Cancers (including chemo and radiation therapies)
    - Peripheral artery disease (PAD)
    - Cardiac arrest

Likewise, certain intellectual and developmental disabilities, such as ASDs, may benefit from rehabilitation medicine in the form of occupational or physical therapy or other rehabilitation services.

These are but a few examples, and many of them fall outside the research portfolio of the *Eunice Kennedy Shriver* National Institute of Child Health and Human Development (NICHD) and National Center for Medical Rehabilitation Research (NCMRR). In general, though, any person might need care related to rehabilitation medicine at some point in her or his life, for a variety of reasons.

Secondary Conditions

Many people who experience the disorders listed above also face their secondary effects—problems that are not necessarily part of the main diagnosis, but that can also have an impact on patients' health, independence, and the quality of life (QOL).

Rehabilitation medicine may include treatments for these and other secondary symptoms:

- Muscle atrophy (wasting), blood clots or circulation issues, obesity, or other problems resulting from disuse
- Problems caused by overuse of prosthetics or medical devices
- Ulcers, bedsores, or other problems with skin integrity
- Local or widespread infections or sepsis
- Injuries resulting from falls
- Problems with balance or vision
- High blood pressure, diabetes, and other conditions
- Bladder and bowel problems
- Breathing problems, including those related to mechanical ventilation
- Emotional or cognitive difficulties, such as anger, depression, or difficulty controlling emotions or behavior

If not addressed in a timely manner, many of these secondary conditions can become serious, some of them fatal.

WHAT TYPES OF ACTIVITIES ARE INVOLVED WITH REHABILITATION MEDICINE?

Rehabilitation medicine uses many kinds of assistance, therapies, and devices to improve function. The type of rehabilitation a person receives depends on the condition causing impairment, the bodily function that is affected, and the severity of the impairment.

The following are some common types of rehabilitation:

- **Cognitive-rehabilitation therapy (CRT)** involves relearning or improving skills, such as thinking, learning, memory, planning, and decision-making that may have been lost or affected by brain injury.

- **Occupational therapy** helps a person carry out daily life tasks and activities in the home, workplace, and community.
- **Pharmacorehabilitation** involves the use of drugs to improve or restore physical or mental function.
- **Physical therapy** involves activities and exercises to improve the body's movements, sensations, strength, and balance.
- **Rehabilitative/assistive technology** refers to tools, equipment, and products that help people with disabilities move and function. This technology includes (but is not limited to):
  - Orthotics, which are devices that aim to improve movement and prevent contracture in the upper and lower limbs. For instance, pads inserted into a shoe, specially fitted shoes, or ankle or leg braces can improve a person's ability to walk. Hand splints and arm braces can help the upper limbs remain supple and unclenched after a spinal cord injury.
  - Prosthetics, which are devices designed to replace a missing body part, such as an artificial limb
  - Wheelchairs, walkers, crutches, and other mobility aids
  - Augmentative/alternative communication (AAC) devices, which aim to either make a person's communication more understandable or take the place of a communication method. They can include electronic devices, speech-generating devices, and picture boards.
  - Hearing aids and cochlear implants
  - Retinal prostheses, which can restore useful vision in cases in which it has been lost due to certain degenerative eye conditions
  - Telemedicine and telerehab technologies, which are devices or software to deliver care or monitor conditions in the home or community
  - Rehabilitation robotics
  - Mobile apps to assist with speech/communication, anxiety/stress, memory, and other functions or symptoms
- **Recreational therapy (RT)** helps improve symptoms and social and emotional well-being through arts and

crafts, games, relaxation training, and animal-assisted therapy.

- **Speech and language therapy (SLT)** aims to improve impaired swallowing and movement of the mouth and tongue, as well as difficulties with the voice, language, and talking.
- **Surgery** includes procedures to correct a misaligned limb or to release a constricted muscle, skin grafts for burns, insertion of chips into the brain to assist with limb or prosthetic movement, and placement of skull plates or bone pins.
- **Vocational rehabilitation (VR)** aids in building skills for going to school or working at a job.
- **Music or art therapy** can specifically aid in helping people express emotion, in cognitive development, or in helping to develop social connectedness.

These services are provided by a number of different healthcare providers and specialists, including (but not limited to):

- Physiatrists (also called "rehabilitation physicians")
- Occupational therapists
- Physical therapists
- Cognitive rehabilitation therapists
- Gait and clinical movement specialist
- Rehabilitation technologists
- Speech therapists
- Audiologists
- Orthopedists/surgeons
- Neurologists
- Psychiatrists/psychologists
- Biomedical engineers
- Rehabilitation engineers

Chapter 29 | Spirituality in Psychiatric Rehabilitation

WHAT IS SPIRITUALITY? IS IT THE SAME AS RELIGION?

Spirituality is a broad concept with many definitions. Entire books have been written on the subject. Spirituality often involves the following:

- Determining what gives you a sense of meaning in life
- Connecting with something "bigger than us"

Religion and spirituality are discussed together, but they are not the same. Religion is a system of beliefs and practices that is often defined by a specific community or social group. Examples of major religions include Christianity, Islam, Judaism, and Hinduism. Religion may include spirituality. But, spirituality does not have to involve religion. People of the same religion may also experience spirituality in different ways.

Spirituality is our experience of how we relate to whatever is greater than ourselves and gives meaning to our lives. It is an experience unique to each person. At the same time, it also involves how we are connected to one another.

WHAT DOES SPIRITUALITY HAVE TO DO WITH HEALTH?

Research has found that religion and spirituality may affect a range of health issues.

This chapter contains text excerpted from the following sources: Text beginning with the heading "What Is Spirituality? Is It the Same as Religion?" is excerpted from "An Introduction to Spirit and Soul for Whole Health," U.S. Department of Veterans Affairs (VA), May 11, 2018; Text beginning with the heading "Spirituality/Religion in the Lives of People with Behavioral Health Disorders" is excerpted from "Talking about Spiritual and Religious Factors in Wellness," Substance Abuse and Mental Health Services Administration (SAMHSA), September 16, 2017.

- **Physical health.** People who attend weekly services with a supportive community have longer life spans. Research has found that religious people smoke less, exercise more, eat more healthy foods, and engage in less risky sexual practices, on average.
- **Mental health.** Spirituality can mean building meaning and connection. Meaning and connection are central to mental health. Having them can build optimism and reduce depression, anxiety, and posttraumatic stress.

Spirituality can help individuals manage problems, such as chronic pain, heart disease, diabetes, arthritis, and stroke. For example, having a spiritual practice (like praying or working with forgiveness) can help people tolerate pain and function better. Spirituality can give people more strength to handle stress, loss, and the effects of war.

WHAT ARE SOME WAYS TO HAVE A SPIRITUAL CONNECTION?

Spirituality can take a variety of different forms. Consider the six examples of spiritual connection described below. Do any of them resonate with you? These are just some ways to think about how we experience spirituality. You may find you relate to more than one.

1. **Connection to a higher power.** This may involve a relationship with a higher power, such as God, as taught by a specific religion.
2. **Connection to humankind.** This may involve love, being kind and serving other people.
3. **Connection to nature.** This might include the wonder you feel when walking in the woods, watching a sunrise, or listening to the ocean waves.
4. **Connection to life experience.** This may include what we learn through our life events and stories.
5. **Connection to the cosmos.** This might include feeling the vastness of the universe, for example, while looking at a sky full of stars.
6. **Connection to the mystery.** This may involve feeling peace with the fact that there is much that we simply cannot know.

This may involve allowing space for what we do not fully understand.

HOW CAN I EXPLORE MY SPIRITUALITY AND HOW IT CONNECTS TO MY HEALTH?

To start with, consider the following questions. If you like, take a few minutes to write down your responses.

- What gives me a sense of meaning and purpose?
- What really matters to me in life?
- What helps me when times are hard? What gives me hope or peace of mind?
- How do my answers to the questions above connect to what I am dealing with in my health right now?
- What does spirituality mean to me? Do I have any spiritual practices that are important in my life?
- Did my experiences in the military affect my spiritual or religious beliefs? If so, how?
- How do I want members of my care team to approach this topic of spirituality and/or religion? Do I prefer that they bring it up, or rather they did not?

How you answer the above questions can help guide you with creating your personal health plan. There may be aspects that evolve and change over time, or remain more constant. Thinking about what is most important to you and how that relates to your health is central to Whole Health.

WHO ON MY CARE TEAM CAN SUPPORT ME IN EXPLORING SPIRITUALITY AND HEALTH?

Chaplains. Chaplains are important members of the Whole Health team. They are available in the United States Department of Veterans Affairs (VA) facilities 24 hours a day. Chaplains receive extensive training to work with people from diverse backgrounds with a variety of spiritual needs. They can provide valuable support to you, as well as to friends and family.

Doctors and nurses. Communicating with your doctors and nurses about what is important to you can help them better understand you as a person. This can be helpful as you work together to reach your health goals. This may include topics ranging from starting a new medication to planning for end-of-life care.

Mental-health providers. Spiritual health and mental health are closely joined. Talking openly about spirituality may help you learn ways to cope with stress and recover from mental illness.

SPIRITUALITY/RELIGION IN THE LIVES OF PEOPLE WITH BEHAVIORAL-HEALTH DISORDERS

There are a number of reasons why providers should consider talking about spirituality with individuals with behavioral health disorders. Most importantly, studies have shown that individuals with higher spirituality and religiosity levels had an 18 percent reduction in mortality rates.

Symptom Management

Individuals who identify as being religious or spiritual report lower rates of psychiatric conditions, such as depression and anxiety. Not only that, individuals who identify as being religious or spiritual report experience improved health outcomes with chronic conditions such and cardiovascular disease (CVD) and type 2 diabetes, which decreases the risk of premature mortality.

Spirituality and Recovery from Serious Mental Illness

Spirituality/religion is an important part of recovery for individuals with serious mental illness (SMI), and many persons would like treatment providers to be made aware of their spiritual beliefs and have this information considered as a part of their treatment planning. To date, the systematic research published in the mental-health literature does not support the argument that religious involvement usually has an adverse effect on mental health and recovery. Rather in general, studies find that religious involvement is related to better coping with stress and less depression, suicide, anxiety, and substance abuse.

Spirituality and Social Support

A significant number of individuals living with psychiatric disabilities report that they have used religion to help them cope. Religious beliefs can provide a sense of meaning and purpose during difficult life circumstances. Unlike many other coping resources, religion is available to anyone at any time, regardless of financial, social, physical, or mental circumstances. Accessing religion can also create opportunities for building support networks, which may be helpful in dealing with stressors individuals living with behavioral health conditions encounter.

Spirituality and Culture

Cultural factors may influence how individuals seek support and access services. For example, individuals experiencing a behavioral health crisis may be more likely to seek support from faith-based organizations. Consequently, it is important to consider religious and faith-based organizations as valued partners. In other words, considering cultural factors such as spirituality/religion can improve engagement and retention.

STRATEGIES FOR TALKING ABOUT SPIRITUALITY/RELIGION WITH INDIVIDUALS WITH SERIOUS MENTAL ILLNESS

Focus on Meaning

As noted earlier, people may use terms such as spirituality and religion interchangeably. Relying on a particular definition may not be the most successful strategy for engaging individuals with serious mental illness. However, engaging people in conversations about the strategies they use to find a sense of meaning and purpose in life and maintain a sense of hope when faced with adversity (overlapping concepts in spirituality, religion, and faith) can create an opportunity for more open dialogue between individuals being served and providers.

Make Use of Existing Resources

Tools such as cultural activation prompts (CAPs) can help. Created by the Nathan Kline Institute Center of Excellence in Culturally Competent Mental Health, CAPs is a tool for promoting cultural activation. It includes a list of 15 cues for consumers to use to convey information to caregivers on what culturally matters to them in receiving care. Through the use of CAPs, individuals receiving services can learn strategies for starting a cultural conversation with their caregivers and providers, including but not limited to their religious/spiritual beliefs. Providers can explore the CAPs, too, and actively work to integrate the tool into service provision.

Be Understanding and Communicative

When talking with the individuals you serve about spirituality, it is important to be understanding. Understanding entails knowing that the spiritual beliefs of the individual you are working with may not be in alignment with your own, while also understanding the myriad of different belief systems that exist. Not only are there a number of belief systems, religions, and faiths, but people exist at different developmental stages of their own spiritual journeys. You may meet an individual who has never considered spiritual wellness as a component of their well-being, whereas another may be a lifetime follower of a particular faith. Be mindful and understanding of these differences and strive to make recommendations or suggestions that meet the individual where they are. This communication can help foster a sense of inclusion. Even if you do not share the same beliefs as the individual you are working with, listen to them share and cooperate to make relevant treatment plans or goals for achieving optimal health and well-being. Clinicians need to be aware of the religious and spiritual activities of the individuals they serve and appreciate their value as a resource for healthy mental and social functioning.

Chapter 30 | Psychotherapies

"Psychotherapy" (sometimes called "talk therapy") is a term for a variety of treatment techniques that aim to help a person identify and change troubling emotions, thoughts, and behavior. Most psychotherapy takes place with a licensed and trained mental-healthcare professional and a patient meeting one on one or with other patients in a group setting.

Someone might seek out psychotherapy for different reasons:

- You might be dealing with severe or long-term stress from a job or family situation, the loss of a loved one, or relationship or other family issues. Or you may have symptoms with no physical explanation: changes in sleep or appetite, low energy, a lack of interest or pleasure in activities that you once enjoyed, persistent irritability, or a sense of discouragement or hopelessness that would not go away.
- A health professional may suspect or have diagnosed a condition such as depression, bipolar disorder, posttraumatic stress disorder (PTSD), or other disorders and recommended psychotherapy as a first treatment or to go along with medication.
- You may be seeking treatment for a family member or child who has been diagnosed with a condition affecting mental health and for whom a health professional has recommended treatment.

An exam by your primary-care practitioner can ensure there is nothing in your overall health that would explain your or a loved one's symptoms.

This chapter includes text excerpted from "Psychotherapies," National Institute of Mental Health (NIMH), November 2016. Reviewed October 2019.

WHAT TO CONSIDER WHEN LOOKING FOR A THERAPIST

Therapists have different professional backgrounds and specialties. There are resources at the end of this material that can help you find out about the different credentials of therapists and resources for locating therapists.

There are many different types of psychotherapy. Different therapies are often variations on an established approach, such as cognitive-behavioral therapy (CBT). There is no formal approval process for psychotherapies as there is for the use of medications in medicine. For many therapies, however, research involving large numbers of patients has provided evidence that treatment is effective for specific disorders. These "evidence-based therapies" have been shown in research to reduce symptoms of depression, anxiety, and other disorders.

The particular approach a therapist uses depends on the condition being treated and the training and experience of the therapist. Also, therapists may combine and adapt elements of different approaches.

One goal of establishing an evidence base for psychotherapies is to prevent situations in which a person receives therapy for months or years with no benefit. If you have been in therapy and feel you are not getting better, talk to your therapist, or look into other practitioners or approaches. The object of therapy is to gain relief from symptoms and improve the quality of life (QOL).

Once you have identified one or more possible therapists, a preliminary conversation with a therapist can help you get an idea of how the treatment will proceed and whether you feel comfortable with the therapist. Rapport and trust are important. Discussions in therapy are deeply personal and it is important that you feel comfortable and trusting with the therapist and have confidence in her or his expertise. Consider asking the following questions:

- What are the credentials and experience of the therapist? Does she or he have a specialty?
- What approach will the therapist take to help you? Does she or he practice a particular type of therapy? What can the therapist tell you about the rationale for the therapy and the evidence base?

- Does the therapist have experience in diagnosing and treating the age group (for example, a child) and the specific condition for which treatment is being sought? If a child is a patient, how will parents be involved in treatment?
- What are the goals of therapy? Does the therapist recommend a specific time frame or the number of sessions? How will progress be assessed and what happens if you (or the therapist) feel you are not starting to feel better?
- Will there be homework?
- Are medications an option? How will medications be prescribed if the therapist is not an M.D.?
- Are our meetings confidential? How can this be assured?

Psychotherapies and Other Treatment Options

Psychotherapy can be an alternative to medication or can be used along with other treatment options, such as medications. Choosing the right treatment plan should be based on a person's individual needs and medical situation and under a mental-health professional's care.

Even when medications relieve symptoms, psychotherapy and other interventions can help a person address specific issues. These might include self-defeating ways of thinking, fears, problems with interactions with other people, or dealing with situations at home and at school or with employment.

Elements of Psychotherapy

A variety of different kinds of psychotherapies and interventions have been shown to be effective for specific disorders. Psychotherapists may use one primary approach or incorporate different elements depending on their training, the condition being treated, and the needs of the person receiving treatment.

Here are examples of the elements that psychotherapies can include:

- Helping a person become aware of ways of thinking that may be automatic but are inaccurate and harmful. (An example might be someone who has a low opinion of her or his own abilities.) The therapist helps the person find ways to question these thoughts, understand how they affect

emotions and behavior, and try ways to change self-defeating patterns. This approach is central to CBT
- Identifying ways to cope with stress
- Examining in-depth a person's interactions with others and offering guidance with social and communication skills, if needed
- Relaxation and mindfulness techniques
- Exposure therapy for people with anxiety disorders. In exposure therapy, a person spends brief periods, in a supportive environment, learning to tolerate the distress of certain items, ideas, or imagined scenes cause. Over time the fear associated with these things dissipates
- Tracking emotions and activities and the impact of each on the other
- Safety planning can include helping a person recognize warning signs, and thinking about coping strategies, such as contacting friends, family, or emergency personnel
- Supportive counseling to help a person explore troubling issues and provide emotional support

eHealth

The telephone, Internet, and mobile devices have opened up new possibilities for providing interventions that can reach people in areas where mental-health professionals may not be easily available and can be at hand 24/7. Some of these approaches involve a therapist providing help at a distance, but others—such as web-based programs and cell phone apps—are designed to provide information and feedback in the absence of a therapist.

Some approaches that use electronic media to provide help for mental health-related conditions have been shown by research to be helpful in some situations, others not as yet. The American Psychological Association (APA) has information to consider before choosing online therapy.

It is important to note that, as with all care for conditions affecting mental health, the treatment needs to be appropriate for the condition and the individual. eHealth approaches may be helpful in some situations, including as support with other in-person treatment, but may not be appropriate or effective as a substitute for in-person care.

There is as yet no central resource for information on the effectiveness of health apps. The following links have information on health information technology in general:

- Health IT. How to Keep Your Health Information Private and Secure from the U.S. Department of Health and Human Services (HHS) (www.healthit.gov/sites/default/files/how_to_keep_your_health_information_private_and_secure.pdf
- Understanding mobile apps (www.consumer.ftc.gov/articles/0018-understanding-mobile-apps) from OnGuardOnline.gov

If you are interested in using a mobile app, read the accompanying information, including whether and how the app has been tested. If you are working with a therapist, consult with her or him for help in evaluating the app.

TAKING THE FIRST STEP

The symptoms of mental disorders can have a profound effect on someone's quality of life and ability to function. Treatment can address symptoms as well as assist someone experiencing severe or ongoing stress. Some of the reasons that you might consider seeking out psychotherapy include:

- Overwhelming sadness or helplessness that does not go away
- Serious, unusual insomnia or sleeping too much
- Difficulty focusing on work or carrying out other everyday activities
- Constant worry and anxiety
- Drinking to excess or any behavior that harms self or others
- Dealing with a difficult transition, such as a divorce, children leaving home, job difficulties, or the death of someone close
- Children's behavior problems that interfere with school, family, or peers

Seeking help is not an admission of weakness, but a step towards understanding and obtaining relief from distressing symptoms.

FINDING A THERAPIST

Many different professionals offer psychotherapy. Examples include psychiatrists, psychologists, social workers, counselors, and psychiatric nurses. Information on the credentials of providers is available from the National Alliance on Mental Illness (NAMI).

Your health plan may have a list of mental-health practitioners who participate in the plan. The resources listed there include links to help find reduced-cost treatment. When talking with a prospective therapist, ask about treatment fees, whether the therapist participates in insurance plans, and whether there is a sliding scale for fees according to income.

The following professional organizations have directories or locators on their websites for mental-healthcare practitioners:

- Academy of Cognitive Therapy (ACT)
- Association for Behavioral and Cognitive Therapies (ABCT)
- American Academy of Child & Adolescent Psychiatry (AACAP)
- American Association for Geriatric Psychiatry (AAGP)
- American Psychiatric Association (APA)
- American Psychological Association (APA)
- National Association of Social Workers (NASW)
- National Register of Health Service Psychologists (HSP)
- Society of Clinical Child and Adolescent Psychology (SCCAP)
- Society of Clinical Psychology

National advocacy organizations have information on finding a mental-health professional and sometimes practitioner locators on their websites. Examples include:

- Anxiety and Depression Association of America (ADAA)
- Attention Deficit Disorder Association (ADDA)
- Children and Adults with Attention Deficit Hyperactivity Disorder (CHADD)
- Depression and Bipolar Support Alliance (DBSA)
- International OCD Foundation (IOCDF)
- Mental Health America (MHA)
- National Alliance on Mental Illness (NAMI)

- Treatment and Research Advancements for Borderline Personality Disorder (TARA4BPD)

University or medical school-affiliated programs may offer treatment options. Search on the website of local university health centers for their psychiatry or psychology departments.

You can also go to the website of your state or county government and search for the health department for information on mental health-related programs within your state.

Chapter 31 | Integrated Care for Mental Health

Older adults with serious mental illnesses (SMI), such as schizophrenia, schizoaffective disorder, and bipolar disorder, have more hospitalizations and 4 times greater risk of death at any given age than those without SMI. They are also 3.5 times more likely to live in a nursing home. Despite higher acute and long-term healthcare costs, adults with SMI experience greater barriers to preventive and routine healthcare, and often receive care that is fragmented and inadequate. These disparities highlight a need for effective and sustainable integrated care models designed specifically to support the special healthcare needs among older adults with SMI.

This chapter provides a summary of evidence-based integrated models of care that address the mental and physical health needs of older adults with SMI.

INTEGRATED CARE FOR OLDER ADULTS WITH SERIOUS MENTAL ILLNESS AND MEDICAL COMORBIDITY

What the Researchers Found

Psychosocial Skills Training

Three group-based programs have research evidence of effectiveness in improving psychosocial skills among older adults with SMI:

1. Helping Older People Experience Success (HOPES) program
2. Functional Adaptation Skills Training (FAST) program
3. Cognitive-Behavioral Social Skills Training (CBSST) program

This chapter contains text excerpted from the following sources: Text in this chapter begins with excerpts from "Integrated Care for Older Adults with Serious Mental Illness and Medical Comorbidity: Evidence-Based Models and Future Research Directions," Administration for Community Living (ACL), May 17, 2019; Text beginning with the heading "Integrated Care" is excerpted from "Integrated Care," National Institute of Mental Health (NIMH), February 2017.

These programs range from 12 weeks CBSST to 12 months HOPES; an integrated health management component of HOPES is delivered by a registered nurse. Common features of all three are that they are group-based, provide accommodations for people with physical or cognitive disabilities, and use age-appropriate cognitive-behavioral principles and skills training techniques to meet the specific needs of older adults with SMI.

Integrated Illness Management and Recovery

Three interventions have been shown to be effective in improving chronic disease self-management among adults with SMI:

1. Health and Recovery Peer (HARP) program,
2. Targeted Training in Illness Management (TTIM), and
3. Integrated Illness Management and Recovery (I-IMR).

The HARP program consists of 6 peer specialist-led sessions and was adapted from the widely-disseminated Chronic Disease Self-Management Program (CDSMP). TTIM is also a group-based and is led by a peer and a nurse educator. This 12-week program blends social support with diabetes and mental-health psychoeducation and goal setting. IIMR combines 4 evidence-based psychosocial interventions—psychoeducation, which improves knowledge about mental illness management; behavioral tailoring which improves medication adherence; coping skills training, which reduces distress related to symptoms; and relapse prevention training.

Behavioral Health Homes

In contrast to the extensive research on integrating mental healthcare in primary care settings, little research has studied colocating primary care within mental-health settings. Three randomized controlled trials (RCTs) that assessed the impact of behavioral health homes on adults with SMI and medical comorbidity were identified. A 2001 study evaluated the effectiveness of colocating primary care services in Veterans Affairs (VA) hospital's mental-health clinics. After 12 months, veterans who received care in this colocated clinic received, on average, more preventive services and self-reported better physical health functioning. The Primary Care Access, Referral and Evaluation (PCARE) intervention involved a nurse care manager, located at a community mental-health center, who coordinated care with medical providers and used motivational interviewing to enhance patient activation, promote self-management and health advocacy skills. In an RCT, after 12 months, patients who received PCARE had more primary care visits and greater reduction in 10-year risk of cardiovascular disease (CVD), compared to those receiving usual care. The 2017 Health Outcomes Management and Evaluation (HOME) study compared outcomes among patients receiving primary care through a behavioral health home to those who received usual care, and found that behavioral health home patients had higher preventive service uptake and better quality of cardiometabolic care, but showed no clinically significant difference in blood pressure, cholesterol, blood glucose, or 10-year cardiovascular risk.

Key Findings

- Social skills training interventions are associated with improved social functioning and independent community living among older adults with serious mental illness.
- Illness self-management programs can improve the management of either psychiatric or medical disorder among older adults with serious mental illness—but integrated interventions that address both are scarce.
- Integrated health homes have the potential to increase access to preventive care and improve the quality of care for chronic medical conditions but inconsistently achieve clinically significant results.

INTEGRATED CARE

Integrated Care combines primary healthcare and mental healthcare in one setting. There are many ways to integrate care, and they may go by different names, including "Collaborative Care" or "Health Homes." This is an important model of care because:

- Primary care settings, such as a doctor's office, provide about half of all mental healthcare for common psychiatric disorders.
- Adults with serious mental illnesses and substance-use disorders (SUDs) also have higher rates of chronic physical illnesses and die earlier than the general population.

- People with common physical health conditions also have higher rates of mental-health challenges.

Providing Integrated Care helps patients and their providers. It blends the expertise of mental health, substance use, and primary care clinicians, with feedback from patients and their caregivers. This creates a team-based approach where mental healthcare and general medical care are offered in the same setting. Coordinating primary care and mental healthcare in this way can help address the physical health challenges of people with serious mental illnesses.

WHY IS IT IMPORTANT?

Addressing the whole person and her or his physical and behavioral health is essential for positive health outcomes and cost-effective care. Many people may not have access to mental healthcare or may prefer to visit their primary healthcare provider. Although most primary care providers can treat mental disorders, particularly through medication, that may not be enough for some patients. Historically, it has been difficult for a primary care provider to offer effective, high-quality mental healthcare when working alone. Combining mental-health services/expertise with primary care can reduce costs, increase the quality of care, and, ultimately, save lives.

Addressing Physical and Behavioral Health

Untreated or undertreated mental illnesses have serious consequences. People with severe mental illness often die 13 to 30 years earlier than the general population from medical conditions that could have been treated by a primary care provider.

Treating Children

Most children with mental-health conditions are treated in a primary care setting instead of a specialized mental-health setting. About half of all mental-health disorders begin by age 14. Accurate diagnoses and quality care are vital in a primary care setting.

Treating Adults

Adults are also more likely to be seen in a primary care setting than within a mental-health system. Primary-care providers deliver half of the mental healthcare for common conditions, such as anxiety, attention deficit hyperactivity disorder (ADHD), depression, behavioral challenges, and substance use. Yet, people with mental illnesses who are treated in a primary care setting are less likely to receive effective behavioral healthcare. For example, 75 percent of adult patients with depression see primary care providers, but only half are accurately diagnosed. When a referral is made to a mental health provider, only about half of patients follow through with making an appointment. As a result, many behavioral health challenges go undetected, undertreated, and/or untreated.

HOW DOES IT WORK?

Integrated Care meets all of a patient's health needs in one setting. It can be delivered in multiple ways depending on who is providing the care, what type of care is being provided, where the care is taking place, and how services are being coordinated. Integration can take place in behavioral health, primary care, specialty clinics, and home health settings.

There are different levels of service integration. The Substance Abuse and Mental Health Service Administration (SAMHSA) designed a framework to help healthcare providers plan and support an integrated system. That framework has three main categories:

- Coordinated Care, which concentrates on communication
- Colocated Care, which focuses on physical proximity
- Integrated Care, which emphasizes practice change

Within each category, there are varying degrees of collaboration between care providers. These levels range from minimal to full integration. Minimal integration is when medical and mental-healthcare providers work in separate facilities, have separate systems, and rarely communicate. Full integration involves a single health system's medical and mental-healthcare providers working simultaneously to treat a patient's behavioral and medical needs with shared medical record access.

The following are examples of Integrated Care programs:

Collaborative Care

A team-based Collaborative Care program adds two new types of services to usual primary care—behavioral healthcare management and consultations with a mental-health specialist.

The behavioral healthcare manager becomes part of the patient's treatment team and helps the primary care provider to evaluate the patient's mental health. If the patient receives a diagnosis of a mental-health disorder and wants treatment, the care manager, primary care provider, and patient work together to develop a treatment plan. This plan may include medication, psychotherapy, or other appropriate options.

Later, the care manager reaches out to see if the patient likes the plan, is following the plan, and if the plan is working or if changes are needed. The care manager and the primary care provider also regularly review the patient's status and care plan with a mental health specialist, such as a psychiatrist or psychiatric nurse, to be sure the patient is getting the best treatment options and improving.

Patient-Centered Medical Home

Another Integrated Care model is the patient-centered medical home (PCMH). PCMH involves coordinating a patient's overall healthcare needs at any age. Patients play active roles in their healthcare. Providers coordinate all aspects of preventive, acute, and chronic needs of patients using the best available evidence and appropriate technology.

As a result of the Affordable Care Act (ACA), health homes were established for individuals on Medicaid with chronic conditions including mental-health and SUDs, asthma, diabetes, heart disease, and obesity. Health homes are team-based with a whole-person approach with specific emphasis on integrating behavioral health and primary care. Health homes provide comprehensive care management, coordination, and follow-up. They also offer patient and family support, referrals to community and support services, and health promotion.

Hub-Based Systems

Found mostly in the child mental health world, hub-based systems modeled on the Massachusetts Child Psychiatry Access Project (MCPAP) provide primary care providers with immediate telephone consultations with a child psychiatrist. Case management and face-to-face evaluations are also available for complicated cases.

Four Quadrant Model

The Four Quadrant Model is a way to measure an organization's level of integration.

The Four Quadrant Clinical Integration Model describes integration levels in terms of primary care and behavioral healthcare complexity and risk. The location, types of providers, and services vary depending on the complexity of patients' conditions.

For instance, individuals with mild-to-moderate physical and/or behavioral health challenges may be best cared for in a primary care setting with integrated behavioral health providers. For patients with complex general medical conditions as well as mild-to-moderate behavioral health disorders, a medical specialty setting with integrated behavioral health providers may be appropriate. Those with severe behavioral challenges as well as medical conditions may receive the most comprehensive care in a specialty behavioral health center with integrated general medical providers, or health home.

Pediatric versus Adult Integrated Care

Pediatric Integrated Care differs from adult Integrated Care in three main ways:

- There is an increased sensitivity to how children are developing, both mentally and emotionally
- Families play an important role
- Treatment emphasizes coping and adjustment techniques in addition to standard care

The general principles of Integrated Care apply to adults as well as children and adolescents, but work with developing youth and their families is often different from the work with adults with complex medical illnesses. In addition, ongoing evaluation for intellectual disability and developmental delays will be emphasized in pediatric evaluations.

Chapter 32 | **Mental-Health Crisis**

Section 32.1 | Crisis Assistance

This section includes text excerpted from "Practice Guidelines—Core Elements in Responding to Mental-Health Crises," Substance Abuse and Mental Health Services Administration (SAMHSA), 2009. Reviewed October 2019.

Adults, children, and older adults with a serious mental illness or emotional disorder often lead lives characterized by recurrent, significant crises. These crises are not the inevitable consequences of mental disability, but rather represent the combined impact of a host of additional factors, including lack of access to essential services and supports, poverty, unstable housing, coexisting substance use, other health problems, discrimination, and victimization.

Homelessness, police contact, institutionalization, and other adverse events are in themselves crises, and may also contribute to further crises. The statistics below paint a sobering picture of how crises affect the lives of people who have mental or emotional disabilities:

- From one third to one-half of homeless people have a severe psychiatric disorder.
- Approximately 7 percent of all police contacts in urban settings involve a person believed to have a mental illness.
- The likelihood of mental illness among people confined in state prisons and local jails is three to four times higher than in the general population and, compared with other inmates, it is at least twice as likely that these individuals will be injured during their incarceration.
- About 6 percent of all hospital emergency department visits involve mental-health emergencies.
- Due to a lack of available alternatives, 79 percent of hospital emergency departments report having to "board" psychiatric patients who are in crisis and in need of inpatient care, sometimes for 8 hours or longer.
- Almost 1 in 10 individuals discharged from a state psychiatric hospital will be readmitted within 30 days; more than 1 in 5 will be readmitted within 180 days.

- About 90 percent of adult inpatients in state psychiatric hospitals report histories of trauma.
- About three-quarters of youth in the juvenile justice system report mental-health problems and 1 in 5 has a serious mental disorder.
- Mothers with serious mental illnesses are more than 4 times as likely as other mothers to lose custody of their children.
- People with serious mental illnesses (SMI) die, on average, 25 years earlier than the general population.

These statistics are incomplete; they reflect just a sampling of scenarios that, while commonplace, constitute significant life crises for individuals with serious mental illnesses.

Many such individuals experience a cascade of crisis events that place them in more than one of these statistical groups. For instance, readmission to a psychiatric institution—a high probability for adults who have been discharged from a state psychiatric hospital, based on these data—may feature a series of crisis events for the individual: the psychiatric emergency itself; forcible removal from one's home; being taken into police custody, handcuffed and transported in the back of a police car; evaluation in the emergency department of a general hospital; transfer to a psychiatric hospital; a civil commitment hearing; and so on. And at multiple points in this series of interventions, there is a likelihood that physical restraints, seclusion, involuntary medication or other coercion may be used. Intense feelings of disempowerment are definitional of mental-health crises, yet as the individual becomes the subject of a "disposition" at each juncture, that person may experience a diminishing sense of control.

In the wake of rare but highly publicized tragedies attributed to people with mental illnesses, there is often a temporary surge in political concern about mental-healthcare and expanding crisis interventions. Sadly, the more commonplace crises endured every day by many thousands of adults, older adults, and children with serious mental or emotional problems tend to generate neither media attention nor political concern.

While no one with a mental or emotional disorder is immune from crises, people in the midst of what are termed "serious mental illnesses"—defined as schizophrenia, bipolar disorder, and major depression—may be most reliant on public systems. They also may be at great risk of recurrent crises and interventions that exacerbate their clinical and social problems. These guidelines focus most specifically on individuals with serious mental or emotional problems who tend to encounter an assortment of governmental or publicly funded interveners when they are in crisis. Nevertheless, the values, principles, and strategies embedded in the guidelines that follow are applicable to all individuals with mental-healthcare needs, across populations and service settings.

Individuals whose diagnoses do not fit "serious mental illnesses" may be vulnerable to serious mental-health crises that can have devastating outcomes. Interventions on their behalf are more likely to occur within the private healthcare sector, which mirrors public mental-health systems' problems in providing early and meaningful access to help. Within these parallel systems, crisis services are provided in a broad array of settings that ultimately will require translation of the guidelines presented here into specific protocols that break cycles of crises and advance the prospects of recovery for people with mental illnesses.

WHAT IT MEANS TO BE IN A MENTAL-HEALTH CRISIS

Too often, public systems respond as if a mental-health crisis and danger to self or others were one and the same. In fact, danger to self or others derives from common legal language defining when involuntary psychiatric hospitalization may occur—at best, this is a blunt measure of an extreme emergency. A narrow focus on dangerousness is not a valid approach to addressing a mental-health crisis. To identify crises accurately requires a much more nuanced understanding and a perspective that looks beyond whether an individual is dangerous or immediate psychiatric hospitalization is indicated.

While behaviors that represent an imminent danger certainly indicate the need for some sort of emergency response, these behaviors may well be the culmination of a crisis episode, rather than the episode in its entirety. Situations involving mental-health crises may follow trajectories that include intense feelings of personal distress (e.g., anxiety, depression, anger, panic, hopelessness), obvious changes in functioning (e.g., neglect of personal hygiene, unusual behavior) or catastrophic life events (e.g., disruptions in personal relationships, support systems or living arrangements; loss of autonomy or parental rights; victimization or natural disasters).

Because only a portion of real-life crises may actually result in serious harm to self or others, a response that is activated only when physical safety becomes an issue is often too little, too late or no help at all in addressing the root of the crisis. And a response that does not meaningfully address the actual issues underlying a crisis may do more harm than good.

THE NEED FOR CRISIS STANDARDS

Individuals experiencing mental-health crises may encounter an array of professionals and nonprofessionals trying to intervene and help: family members, peers, healthcare personnel, police, advocates, clergy, educators, and others. The specific crisis response offered is influenced by a number of variables, among them:

- Where the intervention occurs
- At what time of day it occurs
- When it occurs within the course of the crisis episode
- The familiarity of the intervener with the individual or with the type of problem experienced by the individual
- Interveners' training relating to crisis services
- Resources of the mental-health system and the ready availability of services and supports
- Professional, organizational, or legal norms that define the nature of the encounter and the assistance offered

RESPONDING TO A MENTAL-HEALTH CRISIS

Ten essential values are inherent in, appropriate crisis response, regardless of the nature of the crisis, the situations where assistance is offered or the individuals providing assistance:

1. **Avoiding harm.** Sometimes mental-health crises place the safety of the person, the crisis responders or others in jeopardy. An appropriate response establishes physical safety, but it also establishes the individual's psychological safety. For instance, restraints are sometimes used in

situations where there is an immediate risk of physical harm, yet this intervention has inherent physical and psychological risks that can cause injury and even death. Precipitous responses to individuals in mental-health crises—often initiated with the intention of establishing physical safety—sometimes result in harm to the individual. An appropriate response to mental-health crises considers the risks and benefits attendant to interventions and whenever possible employ alternative approaches, such as controlling danger sufficiently to allow a period of "watchful waiting." In circumstances where there is an urgent need to establish physical safety and few viable alternatives to address an immediate risk of significant harm to the individual or others, an appropriate crisis response incorporates measures to minimize the duration and negative impact of interventions used.

2. **Intervening in person-centered ways.** Mental-health crises may be routine in some settings and, perhaps, have even come to be routine for some people with serious mental health or emotional problems. Nevertheless, appropriate crisis assistance avoids rote interventions based on diagnostic labels, presenting complaint or practices customary to a particular setting. Appropriate interventions seek to understand the individual, her or his unique circumstances and how that individual's personal preferences and goals can be maximally incorporated in the crisis response.
3. **Shared responsibility.** An acute sense of losing control over events or feelings is a hallmark of mental-health crises. In fact, research has shown "feeling out of control" to be the most common reason consumers cite for being brought in for psychiatric emergency care. An intervention that is done to the individual—rather than with the individual—can reinforce these feelings of helplessness. One of the principal rationales for person-centered plans is that shared responsibility promotes engagement and better

outcomes. While crisis situations may present challenges to implementing shared, person-centered plans, ultimately an intervention that considers and, to the extent possible, honors an individual's role in crisis resolution may hold long-term benefits. An appropriate crisis response seeks to assist the individual in regaining control by considering the individual an active partner in—rather than a passive recipient of—services.

4. **Addressing trauma.** Crises, themselves, are intrinsically traumatic and certain crisis interventions may have the effect of imposing further trauma—both physical and emotional. In addition, people with serious mental illness have a high probability of having been victims of abuse or neglect. It is essential that once physical safety has been established, the harm resulting from the crisis or crisis response is evaluated and addressed without delay by individuals qualified to diagnose and initiate needed treatment. There is also a dual responsibility relating to the individual's relevant trauma history and vulnerabilities associated with particular interventions; crisis responders should appropriately seek out and incorporate this information in their approaches, and individuals should take personal responsibility for making this crucial information available (for instance, by executing advance directives).
5. **Establishing feelings of personal safety.** An individual may experience a mental-health crisis as a catastrophic event and, accordingly, may have an urgent need to feel safe. What is regarded as agitated behavior, may reflect an individual's attempts at self-protection, though perhaps to an unwarranted threat. Assisting the individual in attaining the subjective goal of personal safety requires an understanding of what is needed for that person to experience a sense of security (perhaps contained in a crisis plan or personal safety plan previously formulated by the individual) and what interventions increase feelings of vulnerability (for instance, confinement in a room alone). Providing such

assistance also requires that staff be afforded the time to gain an understanding of the individual's needs and latitude to address these needs creatively.

6. **Based on strengths.** Sharing responsibility for crisis resolution means understanding that an individual, even while in crisis, can marshall personal strengths and assist in the resolution of the emergency. Individuals often understand the factors that precipitated a crisis as well as factors that can help ameliorate their impact. An appropriate crisis response seeks to identify and reinforce the resources on which an individual can draw, not only recover from the crisis event but to also help protect against further occurrences.
7. **The whole person.** For individuals who have a mental illness, the psychiatric label itself may shape—even dominate—decisions about which crisis interventions are offered and how they are made available. An individual with a serious mental illness who is in crisis is a whole person, whose established psychiatric disability may be relevant but may—or may not—be immediately paramount. That the individual may have multiple needs and an adequate understanding of the crisis means not being limited by services that are compartmentalized according to healthcare specialty. An individual's emergency may reflect the interplay of psychiatric issues with other health factors. And while the individual is experiencing a crisis that tends to be addressed as a clinical phenomenon, there may also be a host of seemingly mundane, real-world concerns that significantly affect an individual's response: the whereabouts of the person's children, the welfare of pets, whether the house is locked, absence from work, and so on.
8. **The person as a credible source.** Assertions or complaints made by individuals who have been diagnosed with serious mental illness tend to be viewed skeptically by others. Particularly within the charged context of mental-health crises, there may be a presumption that statements made by

these individuals are manifestations of delusional thinking. Consequently, there is a risk that legitimate complaints relating to such matters as a medical illness, pain, abuse or victimization will go unheeded. Even when an individual's assertions are not well-grounded in reality and represent obviously delusional thoughts, the "telling of one's story" may represent an important step toward crisis resolution. For these reasons, an appropriate response to an individual in a mental-health crisis is not dismissive of the person as a credible source of information—factual or emotional—that is important to understand the person's strengths and needs.

9. **Recovery, resilience, and natural supports.** Certain settings, such as hospital emergency departments, may see individuals only transiently, at a point when they are in acute crisis and in a decidedly high-stress environment. Even when not occurring within hospitals, mental-health emergency interventions are often provided in settings that are alien to the individual and the natural supports that may be important parts of her or his daily life. It is important not to lose sight of the fact that an emergency episode may be a temporary relapse and not definitional of the person or that individual's broader life course. An appropriate crisis response contributes to the individual's larger journey toward recovery and resilience and incorporates these values. Accordingly, interventions should preserve dignity, foster a sense of hope, and promote engagement with formal systems and informal resources.
10. **Prevention.** Too often, individuals with serious mental illnesses have only temporary respite between crises. An appropriate crisis response works to ensure that crises will not be recurrent by evaluating and considering factors that contributed to the current episode and that will prevent future relapse. Hence, an adequate crisis response requires measures that address the person's unmet needs, both through individualized planning and by promoting systemic improvements.

Section 32.2 | Suicide Prevention

This section includes text excerpted from "Suicide Prevention," National Institute of Mental Health (NIMH), July 2019.

Suicide is a major public health concern. Over 47,000 people died by suicide in the United States in 2017; it is the tenth leading cause of death overall. Suicide is complicated and tragic, but it is often preventable. Knowing the warning signs for suicide and how to get help can help save lives.

SIGNS AND SYMPTOMS

The behaviors listed below may be signs that someone is thinking about suicide.

- Talking about wanting to die or wanting to kill themselves
- Talking about feeling empty, hopeless, or having no reason to live
- Making a plan or looking for a way to kill themselves, such as searching for lethal methods online, stockpiling pills, or buying a gun
- Talking about great guilt or shame
- Talking about feeling trapped or feeling that there are no solutions
- Feeling unbearable pain (emotional pain or physical pain)
- Talking about being a burden to others
- Using alcohol or drugs more often
- Acting anxious or agitated
- Withdrawing from family and friends
- Changing eating and/or sleeping habits
- Showing rage or talking about seeking revenge
- Taking great risks that could lead to death, such as driving extremely fast
- Talking or thinking about death often
- Displaying extreme mood swings, suddenly changing from very sad to very calm or happy
- Giving away important possessions

- Saying goodbye to friends and family
- Putting affairs in order, making a will

If these warning signs apply to you or someone you know, get help as soon as possible, particularly if the behavior is new or has increased recently.

RISK FACTORS

Suicide does not discriminate. People of all genders, ages, and ethnicities can be at risk. Suicidal behavior is complex, and there is no single cause. Many different factors contribute to someone making a suicide attempt. But people most at risk tend to share specific characteristics. The main risk factors for suicide are:

- Depression, other mental disorders, or substance-abuse disorder
- Certain medical conditions
- Chronic pain
- A prior suicide attempt
- Family history of a mental disorder or substance abuse
- Family history of suicide
- Family violence, including physical or sexual abuse
- Having guns or other firearms in the home
- Having recently been released from prison or jail
- Being exposed to others' suicidal behavior, such as that of family members, peers, or celebrities

Many people have some of these risk factors but do not attempt suicide. It is important to note that suicide is not a normal response to stress. Suicidal thoughts or actions are a sign of extreme distress, not a harmless bid for attention, and should not be ignored.

Often, family and friends are the first to recognize the warning signs of suicide and can be the first step toward helping an at-risk individual find treatment with someone who specializes in diagnosing and treating mental-health conditions.

Suicide is complex. Treatments and therapies for people with suicidal thoughts or actions will vary with age, gender, physical and mental well-being, and with individual experiences.

Identifying People at Risk for Suicide

- **Universal screening.** Research has shown that a three-question screening tool helps emergency room personnel identify adults at risk for suicide. Researchers found that screening all patients–regardless of the reason for their emergency room visit–doubled the number of patients identified as being at risk for suicide. The researchers estimated that suicide-risk screening tools could identify more than three million additional adults at risk for suicide each year.
- **Predicting suicide risk using electronic health records.** Researchers from NIMH partnered with the U.S. Department of Veterans Affairs (VA) and others to develop computer programs that could help predict suicide risk among veterans receiving VA healthcare. Other healthcare systems are beginning to use data from electronic health records to help identify people with suicide risk as well.

TREATMENTS AND THERAPIES

Brief Interventions

- **Safety planning.** Personalized safety planning has been shown to help reduce suicidal thoughts and actions. Patients work with a caregiver to develop a plan that describes ways to limit access to lethal means such as firearms, pills, or poisons. The plan also lists coping strategies and people and resources that can help in a crisis.
- **Follow-up phone calls.** Research has shown that when at-risk patients receive further screening, a Safety Plan intervention, and a series of supportive phone calls, their risk of suicide goes down.

Psychotherapies

Multiple types of psychosocial interventions have been found to help individuals who have attempted suicide. These types of interventions may prevent someone from making another attempt.

- **Cognitive-behavioral therapy (CBT)** can help people learn new ways of dealing with stressful experiences through training. CBT helps individuals recognize their thought patterns and consider alternative actions when thoughts of suicide arise.

- **Dialectical behavior therapy (DBT)** has been shown to reduce suicidal behavior in adolescents. DBT has also been shown to reduce the rate of suicide in adults with a borderline personality disorder, a mental illness characterized by an ongoing pattern of varying moods, self-image, and behavior that often results in impulsive actions and problems in relationships. A therapist trained in DBT helps a person recognize when her or his feelings or actions are disruptive or unhealthy, and teaches the skills needed to deal better with upsetting situations.

Medication

Some individuals at risk for suicide might benefit from medication. Doctors and patients can work together to find the best medication or medication combination, as well as the right dose. Because many individuals at risk for suicide often have a mental illness and substance-use problems, individuals might benefit from medication along with psychosocial intervention.

Clozapine is an antipsychotic medication used primarily to treat individuals with schizophrenia. To date, it is the only medication with a specific U.S. Food and Drug Administration (FDA) indication for reducing the risk of recurrent suicidal behavior in patients with schizophrenia or schizoaffective disorder.

If you are prescribed a medication, be sure you:

- Talk with your doctor or a pharmacist to make sure you understand the risks and benefits of the medications you are taking.
- Do not stop taking a medication without talking to your doctor first. Suddenly stopping a medication may lead to a "rebound" or worsening of symptoms. Other uncomfortable or potentially dangerous withdrawal effects also are possible.
- Report any concerns about side effects to your doctor right away. You may need a change in the dose or a different medication.

- Report serious side effects to the FDA MedWatch Adverse Event Reporting program online or by phone at 800-332-1088. You or your doctor may send a report.

Other medications have been used to treat suicidal thoughts and behaviors, but more research is needed to show the benefit of these options.

Collaborative Care

Collaborative Care has been shown to be an effective way to treat depression and reduce suicidal thoughts. A team-based collaborative care program adds two new types of services to usual primary care: behavioral healthcare management and consultations with a mental-health specialist.

The behavioral healthcare manager becomes part of the patient's treatment team and helps the primary care provider to evaluate the patient's mental health. If the patient receives a diagnosis of a mental-health disorder and wants treatment, the care manager, primary care provider, and patient work together to develop a treatment plan. This plan may include medication, psychotherapy, or other appropriate options.

Later, the care manager reaches out to see if the patient likes the plan, is following the plan, and if the plan is working or if changes are needed to improve the management of the patient's disorders. The care manager and the primary care provider also regularly review the patient's status and care plan with a mental-health specialist, like a psychiatrist or psychiatric nurse, to be sure the patient is getting the best treatment options and improving.

IF YOU KNOW SOMEONE IN CRISIS

Call the National Suicide Prevention Lifeline at 800-273-TALK (800-273-8255), or text the Crisis Text Line (text HELLO to 741741). Both services are free and available 24 hours a day, 7 days a week. The hard of hearing can contact the Lifeline via TTY at 800-799-4889. All calls are confidential. Contact social media outlets directly if you are concerned about a friend's social media updates or dial 911 in an emergency.

The Veterans Crisis Line connects Service members and Veterans in crisis, as well as their family members and friends, with qualified, caring VA's responders through a confidential toll-free hotline, online chat, or text messaging service. Dial 800-273-8255 and press 1 to talk to someone or send a text message to 838255 to connect with a VA responder. You can also start a confidential online chat session at veteranscrisisline.net/get-help/chat.

Chapter 33 | **Health and Well-Being**

Section 33.1 | Components of Health and Well-Being

This section contains text excerpted from the following sources: Text in this section begins with excerpts from "Components of Proactive Health and Well-Being," U.S. Department of Veterans Affairs (VA), September 23, 2014. Reviewed October 2019; Text under the heading "Improving Our Intellectual Wellness" is excerpted from "Creating a Healthier Life, a Step-By-Step Guide to Wellness," Substance Abuse and Mental Health Services Administration (SAMHSA), April 19, 2016. Reviewed October 2019.

Your diet. Your exercise routine. Your sleep patterns. Your relationships and work environment. They are all connected—and they are all important parts of what you can do to enhance your own self-care.

The "Components of Proactive Health and Well-Being" model lays out eight key areas of self-care, illustrating how they fit in with other critical elements of your personal health plan. Improving one area can benefit all other aspects of your life—including your overall physical, mental, and spiritual health and well-being.

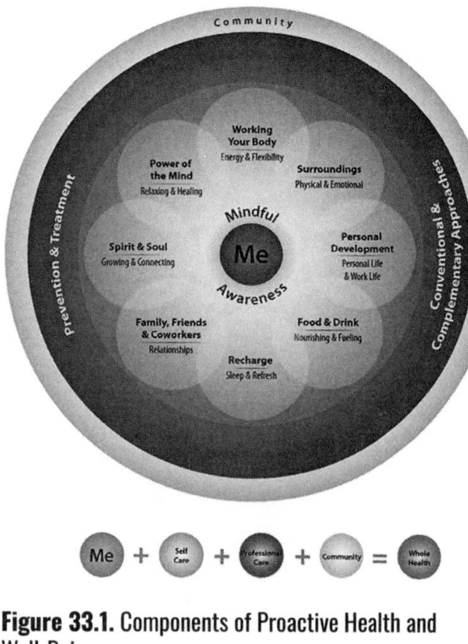

Figure 33.1. Components of Proactive Health and Well-Being

The components of this proactive health and well-being picture will help you think about your overall health. All of the areas in the circle are important. They are all connected. Improving one area can benefit other areas in your life and influence your overall physical, emotional, and mental health and well-being. The human body and mind have tremendous healing abilities and we can strengthen these healing abilities. The inner-circle represents you, your values, and what really matters to you. Being in a state of mindful awareness, of being fully aware and paying attention in the moment, helps you see what matters to you and allows you to make conscious, proactive choices about every aspect of your life and health.

The next area of eight concentric circles represents your self-care. These are the circumstances and choices you make on a daily basis in your everyday life that affect your physical, mental, and spiritual health.

The next ring represents the professional care you receive as part of the prevention and treatment of illnesses or diseases. Professional care may include tests, medications, supplements, surgeries, examinations, treatments, and counseling. This also includes complementary approaches such as acupuncture and mind–body therapies. The outer ring represents the people and groups to whom you are connected reflecting your community.

IMPROVING OUR INTELLECTUAL WELLNESS

The intellectual wellness dimension involves many things that keep your brain active and your intellect expanding. In a broad sense, this dimension can involve looking at different perspectives of an issue and taking each into consideration. Through a number of activities—from learning about current events to organizing game nights in your home or community center—you can broaden your perspective and understand diverse points of view.

Table 33.1. Activities to Improve Intellectual Wellness

Area	Think About	Resources
Personal interests	• Have you considered teaching a class or leading a workshop based on skills, knowledge, or experience you have? • Do you enjoy reading? Might you be interested in books, magazines, blogs, Facebook, etc.? • What would you like to do or learn? Have you considered creative arts such as drawing, pottery, or photography? How about martial arts or learning about nature or about improving your computer skills? • Have you considered inviting a friend, family member, or coworker to attend a lecture, musical performance, or play?	• Find a community group or organization where you could teach a class or a workshop, or lead a discussion. • Consider becoming a member at the local public library to gain access to books, book readings, and other events. • Explore public events in your community by checking out the events section in the newspaper. • Flip through travel books or go online to find places you might enjoy reading about or visiting. • Sign up for a computer class.
Education	• If you are interested in continuing education, are there available classes near you that might lead you to getting a volunteer or paid job or to performing better at a job? • Are you interested in improving your language skills or learning a new language, whether one-onone, through a group class, or via CDs or online resources?	• Check out local college websites for information on classes they offer to the public. • See what kind of skills training—such as writing, sign language, or blogging—might be available at the public library, local congregations, local colleges, or other community organizations.

Table 33.1. continued

Area	Think About	Resources
Brain exercise	• Have you explored thrift shops, libraries, or bookstores for books or DVDs that interest you? • Are you keeping your mind sharp by playing brain games, mind teasers, or fun memory-enhancing games? • Have you read up on current affairs locally, nationally, and internationally lately?	• Subscribe to your local newspaper or pick up a free edition. Many offer sections on subjects that are local, national, and international. • Play crossword puzzles and other games like Sudoku. • Become familiar with websites like Games for the Brain (www.gamesforthebrain. com/).
Conversation	• Do you enjoy taking part in discussions, intellectual conversations, debates, or other ways of gaining an enhanced understanding of issues?	• Befriend people who can stimulate your mind, and get into a discussion with them about topics that interest you.

Section 33.2 | Health and Balance

This section includes text excerpted from "Finding Balance," U.S. Department of Veterans Affairs (VA), April 30, 2018.

Whole Health is an approach to healthcare that empowers and enables you to take charge of your health and well-being and live your life to the fullest. Whole Health starts with you. It is fueled by the power of knowing yourself and what will really work for you in your life. Only you have these insights, this knowledge.

HOW IS BALANCE RELATED TO HEALTH?

It is important to have a balance between different parts of your life, including work, family, free time, and so on. There are many ways to define balance. Some people look at it in terms of how they fit within their community, and others with how they are doing as an individual person. Each of us must define what balance means. For some people, it is a state of mind, or a place of less stress. For others, it involves how much time they spend on different activities. Many people simply say they know when they are or are not balanced. When it comes to Whole Health, the balance might be feeling good about how you are doing in regards to all the different parts of the Circle of Health.

However they define it, people will usually say that balance is an important part of being healthy. Studies confirm this. For example, a study of 25,000 people in 27 countries in Europe looked at how healthy people were based on how they rated the balance between their work lives and their personal lives. People with poor work–life balance had twice the odds of being in poor health.

WHAT MAKES FOR A HEALTHY BALANCE IN LIFE?

There is no simple way to answer that question because everyone is different when it comes to defining balance. You might feel like you must devote a lot of time to work, or you may only feel truly happy when you are with loved ones. Some people are happiest when they are serving others, some when they are able to focus on a skill or talent, and others when they are in nature. Most people care about all of these things, and the trick is to figure out how to give enough time to each one, based on your values. Setting goals for your health can help you to feel more balanced.

Part of working toward Whole Health in your life is to pause and really ask what matters to you. How would you answer the following questions:

- What matters the most to me?
- What is my mission in life?
- What are my dreams and goals?
- What is my calling? My life purpose?

Answers vary. Some people will talk about their faith. Some will talk about important people in their lives, and how they fit in. For others, it may be tied in more with being able to do something they love to do. It might also tie into service, or work, or learning something new. The secret to finding balance is to know what you value, and how to give it regular attention.

WHAT ARE SOME TIPS FOR IMPROVING BALANCE IN YOUR LIFE?

Topics like "Work–Life Balance" have been getting a lot of attention lately because many people find that they are not balanced. The following are some tips to consider, from various experts:

- What we want changes over time. As one couple who does work with burnout put it, a perfectly balanced life is a myth. They talk about balance as something that is always changing because our lives are always changing. It is like walking across a stream on slippery rocks—we have to keep watching and changing our course.
- Focus on reaching one goal at a time. Some people find it easier to focus on details. Instead of saying "I want more balance with my family time and the other parts of my life," they set a goal to have some time with at least one special person in their lives every day. Or they make it a goal to do one thing that is fun every day, or to feel like they reached a goal at work every day. The focus of each day (or a week, or month) can be a different one of those goals.

- Do not wait for a better time to try something, for a different phase of your life. Do not tell yourself, "I will find more balance when I retire" or "I will get to that when the kids are grown" or something like that. We do not know how much time we have, so the balance should be a focus on the present, every day.
- Keep trying, without being too hard on yourself if things are not balanced. It is not about whipping yourself to find balance. In fact, it may be easier to find if you are gentle with yourself. Be careful to have realistic expectations.
- Talk about balance with others. How do your friends and coworkers find balance? What can you learn from them? What can you teach them?

Chapter 34 | Tips for Caring for Someone with a Mental Disability

FOR PARENTS AND CAREGIVERS

As a parent or caregiver, you want the best for your children or other dependents. You may be concerned or have questions about certain behaviors they exhibit and how to ensure they get help.

What to Look For

It is important to be aware of the warning signs that your child may be struggling. You can play a critical role in knowing when your child may need help.

Consult with a school counselor, school nurse, mental-health provider, or another healthcare professional if your child shows one or more of the following behaviors:

- Feeling very sad or withdrawn for more than two weeks
- Seriously trying to harm or kill herself or himself, or making plans to do so
- Experiencing sudden overwhelming fear for no reason, sometimes with a racing heart or fast breathing
- Getting in many fights or wanting to hurt others
- Showing severe out-of-control behavior that can hurt oneself or others
- Not eating, throwing up, or using laxatives to make herself or himself lose weight

This chapter includes text excerpted from "For Parents and Caregivers," MentalHealth.gov, U.S. Department of Health and Human Services (HHS), March 22, 2019.

- Having intense worries or fears that get in the way of daily activities
- Experiencing extreme difficulty controlling behavior, putting herself or himself in physical danger or causing problems in school
- Using drugs or alcohol repeatedly
- Having severe mood swings that cause problems in relationships
- Showing drastic changes in behavior or personality

Because children often cannot understand difficult situations on their own, you should pay particular attention if they experience:

- Loss of a loved one
- Divorce or separation of their parents
- Any major transition—new home, new school, etc.
- Traumatic life experiences, such as living through a natural disaster
- Teasing or bullying
- Difficulties in school or with classmates

What to Do

If you are concerned about your child's behaviors, it is important to get appropriate care. You should:

- Talk to your child's doctor, school nurse, or another healthcare provider and seek further information about the behaviors or symptoms that worry you
- Ask your child's primary care physician if your child needs further evaluation by a specialist with experience in child behavioral challenges.
- Ask if your child's specialist is experienced in treating the problems you are observing
- Talk to your medical provider about any medication and treatment plans

How to Talk about Mental Health

Do you need help starting a conversation with your child about mental health? Try leading with these questions. Make sure you actively listen to your child's response.

- Can you tell me more about what is happening? How you are feeling?
- Have you had feelings like this in the past?
- Sometimes you need to talk to an adult about your feelings. I am here to listen. How can I help you feel better?
- Do you feel like you want to talk to someone else about your problem?
- I am worried about your safety. Can you tell me if you have thoughts about harming yourself or others?

When talking about mental-health challenges with your child, you should:

- Communicate in a straightforward manner
- Speak at a level that is appropriate to a child or adolescent's age and development level (preschool children need fewer details than teenagers)
- Discuss the topic when your child feels safe and comfortable
- Watch for reactions during the discussion and slow down or back up if your child becomes confused or looks upset
- Listen openly and let your child tell you about her or his feelings and worries

FOR FRIENDS AND FAMILY MEMBERS

Anyone can experience mental-health challenges. Friends and family can make all the difference in a person's recovery process.

Supporting a Friend or Family Member

You can help your friend or family member by recognizing the signs of mental-health challenges and connecting them to professional help.

Talking to friends and family about mental-health challenges can be an opportunity to provide information, support, and guidance. Learning about mental-health challenges can lead to:

- Improved recognition of early signs of mental-health challenges
- Earlier treatment
- Greater understanding and compassion

If a friend or family member is showing signs of a mental-health challenge or reaching out to you for help, offer support by:

- Finding out if the person is getting the care that she or he needs and wants—if not, connect her or him to help
- Expressing your concern and support
- Reminding your friend or family member that help is available and that mental-health challenges can be treated
- Asking questions, listening to ideas, and being responsive when the topic of mental-health challenges come up
- Reassuring your friend or family member that you care about her or him
- Offering to help your friend or family member with everyday tasks
- Including your friend or family member in your plans—continue to invite her or him without being overbearing, even if your friend or family member resists your invitations
- Educating other people so they understand the facts about mental-health problems and do not discriminate
- Treating people with mental-health challenges with respect, compassion, and empathy

How to Talk about Mental Health

Do you need help starting a conversation about mental health? Try leading with these questions and make sure to actively listen to your friend or family member's response.

- I have been worried about you. Can we talk about what you are experiencing? If not, who are you comfortable talking to?
- What can I do to help you to talk about issues with your parents or someone else who is responsible and cares about you?
- What else can I help you with?
- I am someone who cares and wants to listen. What do you want me to know about how you are feeling?
- Who or what has helped you deal with similar issues in the past?
- Sometimes talking to someone who has dealt with a similar experience helps. Do you know of others who have experienced these types of problems who you can talk with?

- It seems like you are going through a difficult time. How can I help you to find help?
- How can I help you find more information about mental-health challenges?
- I am concerned about your safety. Have you thought about harming yourself or others?

When talking about mental-health challenges:

- Know how to connect people to help
- Communicate in a straightforward manner
- Speak at a level appropriate to a person's age and development level (preschool children need fewer details as compared to teenagers)
- Discuss the topic when and where the person feels safe and comfortable
- Watch for reactions during the discussion and slow down or back up if the person becomes confused or looks upset

Sometimes it is helpful to make a comparison to a physical illness. For example, many people get sick with a cold or the flu, but only a few get really sick with something serious such as pneumonia. People who have a cold are usually able to do their normal activities. However, if they get pneumonia, they will have to take medicine and may have to go to the hospital.

Similarly, feelings of sadness, anxiety, worry, irritability, or sleep problems are common for most people. However, when these feelings get very intense, last for a long period of time, and begin to interfere with school, work, and relationships, it may be a sign of a mental-health challenge. And just like people need to take medicine and get professional help for physical conditions, someone with a mental-health challenge may need to take medicine and/or participate in therapy in order to get better.

Get Help for Your Friend or Family Member

Seek immediate assistance if you think your friend or family member is in danger of harming themselves. You can call a crisis line or the National Suicide Prevention Line at 800-273-TALK (800-273-8255).

If you think your friend or family member is in need of community mental-health services you can find help in your area.

Chapter 35 | Technology and the Future of Mental-Health Treatment

Technology has opened a new frontier in mental-health support and data collection. Mobile devices like cell phones, smartphones, and tablets are giving the public, doctors, and researchers new ways to access help, monitor progress, and increase understanding of mental well-being.

Mobile mental-health support can be very simple but effective. For example, anyone with the ability to send a text message can contact a crisis center. Technology can also be packaged into an extremely sophisticated app for smartphones or tablets. Such apps might use the device's built-in sensors to collect information on a user's typical behavior patterns. If the app detects a change in behavior, it may provide a signal that help is needed before a crisis occurs. Some apps are stand-alone programs that promise to improve memory or thinking skills. Others help the user connect to a peer counselor or to a healthcare professional.

Excitement about the huge range of opportunities has led to a burst of app development. There are thousands of mental-health apps available in iTunes and Android app stores, and the number is growing every year. However, this technology frontier includes a lot of uncertainty. There are very little industry regulation and very little information on app effectiveness, which can lead consumers to wonder which apps they should trust.

This chapter includes text excerpted from "Technology and the Future of Mental Health Treatment," National Institute of Mental Health (NIMH), September 2019.

Before focusing on the state of science and where it may lead, it is important to look at the advantages and disadvantages of expanding mental-health treatment and research into a mobile world.

THE PROS AND CONS OF MENTAL-HEALTH APPS

Experts believe that technology has a lot of potential for clients and clinicians alike. A few of the advantages of mobile care include:

- **Convenience.** Treatment can take place anytime and anywhere (e.g., at home in the middle of the night or on a bus on the way to work) and may be ideal for those who have trouble with in-person appointments.
- **Anonymity.** Clients can seek treatment options without involving other people.
- **An introduction to care.** Technology may be a good first step for those who have avoided mental healthcare in the past.
- **Lower cost.** Some apps are free or cost less than traditional care.
- **Service to more people.** Technology can help mental-health providers offer treatment to people in remote areas or to many people in times of sudden need (e.g., following a natural disaster or terror attack).
- **Interest.** Some technologies might be more appealing than traditional treatment methods, which may encourage clients to continue therapy.
- **24-hour service.** Technology can provide round-the-clock monitoring or intervention support.
- **Consistency.** Technology can offer the same treatment program to all users.
- **Support.** Technology can complement traditional therapy by extending an in-person session, reinforcing new skills, and providing support and monitoring.
- **Objective data collection.** Technology can quantitatively collect information, such as location, movement, phone use, and other information.

This era of mental-health technology offers great opportunities but also raises a number of concerns. Tackling potential problems will be an important part of making sure new apps provide benefits without causing harm. That is why the mental-health community and software developers are focusing on:

- **Effectiveness.** The biggest concern with technological interventions is obtaining scientific evidence that they work and that they work as well as traditional methods.
- **For whom and for what.** Another concern is understanding if apps work for all people and for all mental-health conditions.
- **Privacy.** Apps deal with very sensitive personal information so app makers need to be able to guarantee privacy for app users.
- **Guidance.** There are no industry-wide standards to help consumers know if an app or other mobile technology is proven effective.
- **Regulation.** The question of who will or should regulate mental-health technology and the data it generates needs to be answered.
- **Overselling.** There is some concern that if an app or program promises more than it delivers, consumers may turn away from other, more effective therapies.

TRENDS IN APP DEVELOPMENT

Creative research and engineering teams are combining their skills to address a wide range of mental-health concerns. Some popular areas of app development include:

Self-Management Apps

"Self-management" means that the user puts information into the app so that the app can provide feedback. For example, the user might set up medication reminders, or use the app to develop tools for managing stress, anxiety, or sleep problems. Some software can use additional equipment to track heart rate, breathing patterns, blood pressure, etc., and may help the user track progress and receive feedback.

Apps for Improving Thinking Skills

Apps that help the user with cognitive remediation (improved thinking skills) are promising. These apps are often targeted toward people with serious mental illnesses.

Skill-Training Apps

Skill-training apps may feel more like games than other mental-health apps as they help users learn new coping or thinking skills. The user might watch an educational video about anxiety management or the importance of social support. Next, the user might pick some new strategies to try and then use the app to track how often those new skills are practiced.

Illness Management, Supported Care

This type of app technology adds additional support by allowing the user to interact with another human being. The app may help the user connect with peer support or may send information to a trained healthcare provider who can offer guidance and therapy options. Researchers are working to learn how much human interaction people need for app-based treatments to be effective.

Passive Symptom Tracking

A lot of effort is going into developing apps that can collect data using the sensors built into smartphones. These sensors can record movement patterns, social interactions (such as the number of texts and phone calls), behavior at different times of the day, vocal tone and speed, and more. In the future, apps may be able to analyze these data to determine the user's real-time state of mind. Such apps may be able to recognize changes in behavior patterns that signal a mood episode such as mania, depression, or psychosis before it occurs. An app may not replace a mental-health professional, but it may be able to alert caregivers when a client needs additional attention. The goal is to create apps that support a range of users, including those with serious mental illnesses.

Data Collection

Data collection apps can gather data without any help from the user. Receiving information from a large number of individuals at the same time can increase researchers' understanding of mental health and help them develop better interventions.

RESEARCH VIA SMARTPHONE?

Dr. Patricia Areán's pioneering BRIGHTEN study showed that research via smartphone app is already a reality. The BRIGHTEN study was remarkable because it used technology to both deliver treatment interventions and also to actually conduct the research trial. In other words, the research team used technology to recruit, screen, enroll, treat, and assess participants. BRIGHTEN was especially exciting because the study showed that technology can be an efficient way to pilot test promising new treatments and that those treatments need to be engaging.

A NEW PARTNERSHIP: CLINICIANS AND ENGINEERS

Researchers have found that interventions are most effective when people like them, are engaged and want to continue using them. Behavioral health apps will need to combine the engineers' skills for making an app easy to use and entertaining with the clinician's skills for providing effective treatment options.

Researchers and software engineers are developing and testing apps that do everything from managing medications to teaching coping skills to predict when someone may need more emotional help. Intervention apps may help someone give up smoking, manage symptoms, or overcome anxiety, depression, posttraumatic stress disorder (PTSD), or insomnia. While the apps are becoming more appealing and user-friendly, there still is not a lot of information on their effectiveness.

EVALUATING APPS

There are no review boards, checklists, or widely accepted rules for choosing a mental-health app. Most apps do not have peer-reviewed research to support their claims, and it is unlikely that every mental-health app will go through a randomized, controlled research trial to test effectiveness. One reason is that testing is a slow process and technology evolves quickly. By the time an app has been put through rigorous scientific testing, the original technology may be outdated.

There are no national standards for evaluating the effectiveness of hundreds of mental-health apps that are available. Consumers should be cautious about trusting a program. However, there are a few suggestions for finding an app that may work for you:

- Ask a trusted healthcare provider for a recommendation. Some larger providers may offer several apps and collect data on their use.
- Check to see if the app offers recommendations for what to do if symptoms get worse or if there is a psychiatric emergency.
- Decide if you want an app that is completely automated or an app that offers opportunities for contact with a trained person.
- Search for information on the app developer. Can you find helpful information about her or his credentials and experience?
- Beware of misleading logos. The National Institute of Mental Health (NIMH) has not developed and does not endorse any apps. However, some app developers have unlawfully used the NIMH logo to market their products.
- Search the PubMed database offered by the U.S. National Library of Medicine (NLM). This resource contains articles on a wide range of research topics, including mental-health app development.
- If there is no information about a particular app, check to see if it is based on a treatment that has been tested. For example, research has shown that Internet-based cognitive-behavior therapy (CBT) is as effective as conventional CBT for disorders that respond well to CBT, like depression, anxiety, social phobia, and panic disorder.
- Try it. If you are interested in an app, test it for a few days and decide if it is easy to use, holds your attention, and if you want to continue using it. An app is only effective if keeps users engaged for weeks or months.

WHAT IS NATIONAL INSTITUTE OF MENTAL HEALTH'S ROLE IN MENTAL-HEALTH INTERVENTION TECHNOLOGY?

Between FY2009 and FY2015, NIMH awarded 404 grants totaling 445 million for technology-enhanced mental-health intervention grants. These grants were for studies of computer-based interventions designed to prevent or treat mental-health disorders.

The NIMH staff actively review and evaluate research grants related to technology. These grants focused on:

- Feasibility, efficacy, and effectiveness research
- Technology for disorders, such as schizophrenia, human immunodeficiency virus (HIV), depression, anxiety, autism, suicide, and trauma
- More interventions for cognitive issues, illness management, behavior, and health communication
- Fewer interventions for a personal computer and more interventions for mobile devices
- More engaging ways to deliver therapies or skill development (for example, interactive formats or game-like approaches)
- Real-time (users exchanging information with peers or professionals as needed)
- Active and passive mobile assessment/monitoring

A significant portion of NIMH funding of these types of technologies is through the Small Business Innovation Research (SBIR) and Small Business Technology Transfer (STTR) Programs.

In addition, NIMH created the *National Advisory Mental Health Council Workgroup on Opportunities and Challenges of Developing Information Technologies on Behavioral and Social Science Research* to track and guide the cutting edge of this rapidly-changing area. In 2017, the workgroup released a report reviewing the opportunities for—and the challenges of—using information technologies to study human behaviors relevant to the NIMH mission. NIMH's interest in this area of research was further highlighted in a 2018 notice identifying research on digital health technology to advance the assessment, detection, prevention, treatment, and delivery of services for mental-health conditions as a high-priority area for the Institute.

THE FUTURE: WHAT TYPES OF RESEARCH DOES NATIONAL INSTITUTE OF MENTAL HEALTH EXPECT IN THE FUTURE?

There has been increased interest in:

- Using mobile technology for a wider range of disorders, from mild depression or anxiety to schizophrenia, autism, and suicide
- Developing and refining interventions, instead of adapting existing interventions to work with technologies
- Developing technologies that work on any device
- Incorporating face-to-face contact or remote counseling (phone or online) to provide a balance between technology and the "human touch"

Part 4 | **Protections, Rights, and Benefits**

Chapter 36 | Americans with Disabilities Act

One in three Social Security Disability (SSD) beneficiaries has a mental illness. For many coping with mental illness, the road to finding a job is not easy and commonly takes more than one attempt with help from work incentives, like expedited reinstatement.

The Americans with Disabilities Act (ADA) definition of "disability" includes people with mental illnesses who have a physical or mental impairment that greatly limits one or more major life activities.

The ADA protects people with mental illness by way of:

- **Antidiscrimination rules**—Title I of the ADA blocks private employers from discriminating against suitable people with disabilities—including those with mental illness—when they are applying for jobs. The rule also protects people with disabilities and mental illnesses in situations related to promotions, firing, payment, and other freedoms of employment.
- **Requirements for job accommodations**—Under the ADA, an employer must provide "reasonable accommodations" to qualified employees with disabilities. Reasonable accommodations are changes to a work setting that allow you to perform your job tasks. Accommodations may include supports, such as assistive technology, changes to work settings, or adjusted work schedules.

This chapter contains text excerpted from the following sources: Text in this chapter begins with excerpts from "How the Americans with Disabilities Act (ADA) Protects People with Mental Illness," U.S. Social Security Administration (SSA), May 28, 2015. Reviewed October 2019; Text under the heading "Which Psychiatric Disorders Are Considered a Disability?" is excerpted from "Sharing the Dream: Is the ADA Accommodating All?" United States Commission on Civil Rights (USCCR), October 15, 2000. Reviewed October 2019.

If you are an employee with mental illness, your employer has to make reasonable accommodations if they know about your condition. Under Title I of the ADA, there are two exceptions to this requirement:

- An employer is not required to provide an accommodation if it will present an "undue hardship" on the business. For example, if accommodations are very costly or would deeply alter the nature of the business.
- An employer may refuse to hire or accommodate an individual who poses a "direct threat" to the health or safety in the workplace. That determination must be based on evidence from a healthcare provider or other source, and not on personal fears and stigmas about mental illness.

Under the ADA, you have a right to request reasonable accommodations to help you succeed in the workplace. Examples of reasonable accommodations for people with mental illnesses include:

- Flexible hours
- Adjusted job tasks
- Leave (paid or unpaid) during periods of illness or hospitalization
- Being assigned a supportive and understanding boss
- Regular guidance and feedback about job performance

For more on job accommodations for people with mental illnesses, visit the Job Accommodation Network (JAN) (askjan.org) or call their free helpline at 800-526-7234 (Voice/TTY).

If you are an employee or job seeker with mental illness, and you believe that you have experienced employment discrimination, you have the right to file an administrative "charge" under Title I of the ADA with the U.S. Equal Employment Opportunity Commission (EEOC). Contact the Commission at 800-669-4000. Social Security beneficiaries who receive Social Security Disability (SSDI) or Supplemental Security Income (SSI) may receive legal advice and services through a program called "Protection and Advocacy for Beneficiaries of Social Security" (PABSS).

You can also find answers to common questions about the ADA and persons with psychiatric disabilities.

Social Security's Ticket to Work (Ticket) program has helped people with mental illnesses find the services and support they need to reach financial independence.

The Ticket program can help people with mental illness create a path to a better financial future. Are you or someone you know receiving disability benefits and want to work? The Ticket program has the resources, supports, and services to help job seekers with disabilities pursue and reach career goals. Call 866-968-7842 or 866-833-2967 (Toll-free TTY) to talk to someone about your situation and how the Ticket program can help you.

WHICH PSYCHIATRIC DISORDERS ARE CONSIDERED A DISABILITY?

The Americans with Disabilities Act (ADA) defines psychiatric disability as a "mental impairment that substantially limits one or more of the major life activities of an individual; a record of impairment; or being regarded as having such an impairment." The U.S. Equal Employment Opportunity Commission's (EEOC) regulations define "mental impairment" to include "any mental or psychological disorder, such as emotional or mental illness." The examples of impairments in psychiatric enforcement guidance include, "major depression, bipolar disorder, anxiety disorders (which include panic disorder, obsessive-compulsive disorder, and posttraumatic stress disorder), schizophrenia, and personality disorders." The psychiatric enforcement guidance further provides that the current edition of the American Psychiatric Association's (APA) *Diagnostic and Statistical Manual of Mental Disorders* (*DSM-IV*) is relevant for identifying these disorders and notes that Congress expressly excluded several specific conditions from ADA's protections.

The EEOC's broad definition of what may constitute an impairment—the *DSM-IV* lists more than 374 psychiatric disorders, three fourth of this alarmed some employers and employment attorneys because, they contend, it muddies employers' ability to correctly identify those individuals entitled to protection under the ADA. Labor attorney James McDonald testified that a listing in the *DSM-IV* should be required and is only a starting point for determining whether a condition is mental impairment. "ADA's legislative history and at least one court decision recognize that Congress intended that only mental disorders as defined in the [*DSM-IV*] may qualify as 'mental impairments' potentially covered by the ADA." Mr. McDonald would narrow the category of impairment because he believes that personality disorders, which are listed in the *DSM-IV*, should be excluded from ADA coverage. The psychiatric enforcement guidance's inclusion of personality disorders as impairments, Mr. McDonald said, "Provides a plethora of new opportunities for problem employees to disguise their misconduct as a disease. Although a nasty or insubordinate employee might not qualify as a person with a disability if his bad attitude is considered in isolation, if his attitude can be linked somehow to a personality disorder, he will be considered to have an "impairment" that may qualify for ADA coverage."

This is problematic, according to Mr. McDonald, because personality disorders are characterized more by aberrant behavior—that many employers would find objectionable—than by disordered thought or mood.

Chapter 37 | **Rights of Students with Hidden Disabilities**

INTRODUCTION TO CIVIL RIGHTS OF STUDENTS WITH HIDDEN DISABILITIES

Section 504 of the Rehabilitation Act of 1973 protects the rights of persons with a disability in programs and activities that receive Federal financial assistance. Section 504 protects the rights not only of individuals with visible disabilities but also those with disabilities that may not be apparent.

Section 504 provides that: "No otherwise qualified individual with a disability in the United States shall, solely by reason of her or his disability, be excluded from the participation in, be denied the benefits of, or be subjected to discrimination under any program or activity receiving Federal financial assistance."

The U.S. Department of Education (ED) enforces Section 504 in programs and activities that receive financial assistance from ED. Recipients of this assistance include public school districts, institutions of higher education, and other state and local education agencies. ED maintains an Office for Civil Rights (OCR), with ten regional offices and a headquarters office in Washington, DC, to enforce Section 504 and other civil rights laws that pertain to recipients of ED funds.

This chapter includes text excerpted from "The Civil Rights of Students with Hidden Disabilities under Section 504 of the Rehabilitation Act of 1973," The U.S. Department of Education (ED), February 1, 2001. Reviewed October 2019.

DISABILITIES COVERED UNDER SECTION 504

The ED Section 504 regulation defines an "individual with a disability" as any person who has a physical or mental impairment which substantially limits one or more major life activities has a record of such an impairment or is regarded as having such an impairment. The regulation further defines a physical or mental impairment as any physiological disorder or condition, cosmetic disfigurement, or anatomical loss affecting one or more of the following body systems: neurological; musculoskeletal; special sense organs; respiratory, including speech organs; cardiovascular; reproductive; digestive; genitourinary; hemic and lymphatic; skin; and endocrine; or any mental or psychological disorder, such as mental retardation, organic brain syndrome, emotional or mental illness, and specific learning disabilities. The definition does not set forth a list of specific diseases and conditions that constitute physical or mental impairments because of the difficulty of ensuring the comprehensiveness of any such list.

The key factor in determining whether a person is considered an "individual with a disability" covered by Section 504 is whether the physical or mental impairment results in a substantial limitation of one or more major life activities. Major life activities, as defined in the regulation, include functions such as caring for one's self, performing manual tasks, walking, seeing, hearing, speaking, breathing, learning, and working.

The impairment must have a material effect on one's ability to perform a major life activity. For example, an individual who has a physical or mental impairment would not be considered a person with a disability if the condition does not in any way limit the individual or only results in some minor limitation. However, in some cases, Section 504 also protects individuals who do not have a disability but are treated as though they do because they have a history of, or have been misclassified as having, a mental or physical impairment that substantially limits one or more major life activities. For example, if you have a history of a disability, but no longer have the condition, or have been incorrectly classified as having such a condition, you too are protected from discrimination under Section 504. Frequently occurring examples of the first group are persons with histories of mental or emotional illness, heart disease, or cancer; of the second group, persons who have been misclassified as mentally retarded. Persons who are not disabled may be covered by Section 504 also if they are treated as if they are a person with a disability, for example, if they are infected with the human immunodeficiency virus.

WHAT ARE HIDDEN DISABILITIES?

Hidden disabilities are physical or mental impairments that are not readily apparent to others. They include such conditions and diseases as specific learning disabilities, diabetes, epilepsy, and allergy. A disability, such as a limp, paralysis, total blindness or deafness is usually obvious to others. But, hidden disabilities such as low vision, poor hearing, heart disease, or chronic illness may not be obvious. Chronic illness involves a recurring and long-term disability, such as diabetes, heart disease, kidney and liver disease, high blood pressure, or ulcers.

Approximately four million students with disabilities are enrolled in public elementary and secondary schools in the United States. Of these 43 percent are classified as a student with a disability, eight percent as emotionally disturbed, and one percent as other health impaired. These hidden disabilities often cannot be readily known without the administration of appropriate diagnostic tests.

THE RESPONSIBILITIES OF U.S. DEPARTMENT OF EDUCATION RECIPIENTS IN PRESCHOOL, ELEMENTARY, SECONDARY, AND ADULT EDUCATION

For coverage under Section 504, an individual with a disability must be "qualified" for service by the school or institution receiving ED funds. For example, the ED Section 504 regulation defines a "qualified disabled person" with respect to public preschool, elementary, secondary, or adult education services, as a person with a disability who is:

- Of an age during which persons without a disability are provided such services
- Of any age during which it is mandatory under state law to provide such services to persons with a disability

- A person for whom a state is required to provide a free appropriate public education under the Individuals with Disabilities education act

Under Section 504 regulation, a recipient that operates a public elementary or secondary education program has a number of responsibilities toward qualified disabled persons in its jurisdiction. These recipients must:

- Undertake annually to identify and locate all unserved disabled children
- Provide a "free appropriate public education" to each student with a disability, regardless of the nature or severity of the disability. This means providing regular or special education and related aids and services designed to meet the individual educational needs of a disabled person as adequately as the needs of a person without a disability are met
- Ensure that each student with a disability is educated with the students without a disability to the maximum extent appropriate to the needs of the disabled
- Establish nondiscriminatory evaluation and placement procedures to avoid the inappropriate education that may result from the misclassification or misplacement of students
- Establish procedural safeguards to enable parents and guardians to participate meaningfully in decisions regarding the evaluation and placement of their children
- Afford disabled children an equal opportunity to participate in nonacademic and extracurricular services and activities

A recipient that operates a preschool education or day care program, or an adult education program may not exclude qualified disabled persons and must take into account their needs of qualified disabled persons in determining the aid, benefits, or services to be provided under those programs and activities.

Students with hidden disabilities frequently are not properly diagnosed. For example, a student with an undiagnosed hearing impairment may be unable to understand much of what a teacher says; a student with a learning disability may be unable to process oral or written information routinely, or a student with an emotional problem may be unable to concentrate in a regular classroom setting. As a result, these students, regardless of their intelligence, will be unable to fully demonstrate their ability or attain educational benefits equal to that of a student without a disability. They may be perceived by teachers and fellow students as slow, lazy, or as discipline problems.

Whether a child is already in school or not, if her or his parents feel the child needs special education or related services, they should get in touch with the local superintendent of schools. For example, a parent who believes her or his child has a hearing impairment or is having difficulty understanding a teacher may request to have the child evaluated so that the child may receive an appropriate education. A child with behavior problems, or one who is doing poorly academically, may have an undiagnosed hidden disability. A parent has the right to request that the school determine whether the child is disabled and whether special education or related services are needed to provide the child with an appropriate education. Once it is determined that a child needs special education or related services, the recipient school system must arrange to provide appropriate services.

THE RESPONSIBILITIES OF U.S. DEPARTMENT OF EDUCATION RECIPIENTS IN POSTSECONDARY EDUCATION

The ED Section 504 regulation defines a qualified individual with a disability for postsecondary education programs as a person with a disability who meets the academic and technical standards requisite for admission to, or participation in, the college's education program or activity.

A college has no obligation to identify students with a disability. In fact, Section 504 prohibits a postsecondary education recipient from making a preadmission inquiry as to whether an applicant for admission is a disabled person. However, a postsecondary institution is required to inform applicants and other interested parties of the availability of auxiliary aids, services, and academic adjustments, and the name of the person designated to coordinate the college's efforts to carry out the requirements of Section 504. After admission (including the period between admission and enrollment), the college may make confidential inquiries as to whether a person has a disability for the purpose of determining whether certain academic adjustments or auxiliary aids or services may be needed.

Many students with hidden disabilities, seeking college degrees, were provided with special education services during their elementary and secondary school years. It is especially important for these students to understand that postsecondary institutions also have responsibilities to protect the rights of students with disabilities. In elementary and secondary school, their school district was responsible for identifying, evaluating, and providing individualized special education and related services to meet their needs. At the postsecondary level, however, there are some important differences. The key provisions of Section 504 at the postsecondary level are highlighted below.

At the postsecondary level, it is the student's responsibility to make her or his disabled condition known and to request academic adjustments. This should be done in a timely manner. A student may choose to make his or her needs known to the Section 504 Coordinator, to an appropriate dean, to a faculty advisor, or to each professor on an individual basis.

A student who requests academic adjustments or auxiliary aids because of a disabling condition may be requested by the institution to provide documentation of the disability and the need for the services requested. This may be especially important to an institution attempting to understand the nature and extent of a hidden disability.

The requested documentation may include the results of medical, psychological, or emotional diagnostic tests, or other professional evaluations to verify the need for academic adjustments or auxiliary aids.

HOW CAN THE NEEDS OF STUDENTS WITH HIDDEN DISABILITIES BE ADDRESSED?

The following examples illustrate how schools can address the needs of their students with hidden disabilities.

- A student with a long-term, debilitating medical problem such as cancer, kidney disease, or diabetes may be given special consideration to accommodate the student's needs. For example, a student with cancer may need a class schedule that allows for rest and recuperation following chemotherapy.
- A student with a learning disability that affects the ability to demonstrate knowledge on a standardized test or in certain testing situations may require modified test arrangements, such as oral testing or different testing formats.
- A student with a learning disability or impaired vision that affects the ability to take notes in class may need a notetaker or tape recorder.
- A student with a chronic medical problem such as kidney or liver disease may have difficulty walking distances or climbing stairs. Under Section 504, this student may require special parking space, sufficient time between classes, or other considerations, to conserve the student's energy for academic pursuits.
- A student with diabetes, which adversely affects the body's ability to manufacture insulin, may need a class schedule that will accommodate the student's special needs.
- An emotionally or mentally ill student may need an adjusted class schedule to allow time for regular counseling or therapy.
- A student with epilepsy who has no control over seizures, and whose seizures are stimulated by stress or tension, may need accommodation for such stressful activities as lengthy academic testing or competitive endeavors in physical education.
- A student with arthritis may have persistent pain, tenderness or swelling in one or more joints. A student experiencing arthritic pain may require a modified physical education program.

Chapter 38 | **Accommodations for Employees with Psychiatric Disabilities**

A psychiatric disability can impact various aspects of an individual's life, including the ability to achieve maximum productivity in the workplace. The National Institute of Mental Health (NIMH) estimates that one in five people will experience a psychiatric disability in their lifetime, and one in four Americans currently knows someone who has a psychiatric disability. It is likely that most employers have at least one employee with a psychiatric disability.

Under the Americans with Disabilities Act (ADA) and other nondiscrimination laws, most employers must provide "reasonable accommodations" to qualified employees with disabilities. Many employers are aware of different types of accommodations for people with physical and communication disabilities, but they may be less familiar with accommodations for employees with disabilities that are not visible, such as psychiatric disabilities. Over the last few years, increasing numbers of employers have expressed a desire and need for information and ideas on accommodations for employees with psychiatric disabilities.

Reasonable accommodations are adjustments to a work setting that make it possible for qualified employees with disabilities to perform the essential functions of their jobs. The majority of accommodations can be made for minimal (if any) cost and a small investment of time and planning. Moreover, effective accommodations can be good for business. They help employees return to work more quickly

This chapter includes text excerpted from "Maximizing Productivity: Accommodations for Employees with Psychiatric Disabilities," Office of Disability Employment Policy (ODEP), U.S. Department of Labor (DOL), April 6, 2006. Reviewed October 2019.

after disability or medical leave, eliminate costs due to lost productivity and can be key to recruiting and retaining qualified employees.

Not all employees with psychiatric disabilities need accommodations to perform their jobs. For those who do, it is important to remember that the process of developing and implementing accommodations is individualized and should begin with input from the employee. Accommodations vary, just as people's strengths, work environments, and job duties vary.

Below are examples of accommodations that have helped employees with psychiatric disabilities to more effectively perform their jobs. The list below does not include all possible accommodations, but it is a good starting point and provides some of the most effective and frequently used workplace accommodations. For example:

- **Flexible workplace**—Telecommuting and/or working from home
- **Scheduling**—Part-time work hours, job sharing, adjustments in the start or end of work hours, compensation time and/or "make up" of missed time
- **Leave**—Sick leave for reasons related to mental health, flexible use of vacation time, additional unpaid or administrative leave for treatment or recovery, leaves of absence and/or use of occasional leave (a few hours at a time) for therapy and other related appointments
- **Breaks**—Breaks according to individual needs rather than a fixed schedule, more frequent breaks and/or greater flexibility in scheduling breaks, provision of backup coverage during breaks, and telephone breaks during work hours to call professionals and others needed for support
- **Other policies**—Beverages and/or food permitted at workstations, if necessary, to mitigate the side effects of medications, on-site job coaches

MODIFICATIONS

- Reduction and/or removal of distractions in the work area
- Addition of room dividers, partitions, or other soundproofing or visual barriers between workspaces to reduce noise or visual distractions

- Private offices or private space enclosures
- Office or workspace location away from noisy machinery
- Reduction of workplace noise that can be adjusted (such as telephone volume).
- Increased natural lighting or full-spectrum lighting
- Music (with headset) to block out distractions

EQUIPMENT OR TECHNOLOGY

- Tape recorders for recording or reviewing meetings and training session
- "White noise" or environmental sound machine
- Handheld electronic organizers, software calendars and organizer programs
- Remote job coaching, laptop computers, personal digital assistants and office computer access via remote locations
- Software that minimizes computerized distractions, such as pop-up screens

JOB DUTIES

- Modification or removal of nonessential job duties or restructuring of the job to include only the essential job functions
- Division of large assignments into smaller tasks and goals
- Additional assistance and/or time for orientation activities, training and learning job tasks and new responsibilities
- Additional training or modified training materials

MANAGEMENT OR SUPERVISION

- Implementation of flexible and supportive supervision style; positive reinforcement and feedback; adjustments in the level of supervision or structure, such as more frequent meetings to help prioritize tasks; and open communication with supervisors regarding performance and work expectations
- Additional forms of communication and/or written and visual tools, including communication of assignments and instructions in the employee's preferred learning style (written, verbal, e-mail, demonstration); creation and

implementation of written tools, such as daily "to-do" lists, step-by-step checklists, written (in addition to verbal) instructions and typed minutes of meetings
- Regularly scheduled meetings (weekly or monthly) with employees to discuss workplace issues and productivity, including annual discussions as part of performance appraisals to assess abilities and discuss promotional opportunities.
- Development of strategies to deal with problems before they arise
- Written work agreements that include any agreed-upon accommodations, long-term and short-term goals, expectations of responsibilities and consequences of not meeting performance standards
- Education of all employees about their right to accommodations
- Relevant training for all employees, including coworkers and supervisory staff

Chapter 39 | Impact of Mental-Health Conditions in the Workplace

Section 39.1 | How Do Mental Health and Chronic Disease Affect Employees and the Workplace?

This section includes text excerpted from "Mental Health and Chronic Diseases," Centers for Disease Control and Prevention (CDC), October 2012. Reviewed October 2019.

ISSUE—HOW DO MENTAL HEALTH AND CHRONIC DISEASE AFFECT DAILY LIFE?

The cost to treat those with chronic diseases is approximately 75 percent of the total national health expenditures. Expenses related to cardiovascular disease alone were estimated to be $503 billion in 2010.

Direct and indirect costs associated with mental health are also costly. The Agency for Healthcare Research and Quality found that in 2006, $57.5 billion was spent on mental-healthcare in the United States. It is estimated that about one-third of those with mental illnesses are employed. One study estimates nearly a quarter of the U.S. workforce (28 million workers aged 18 to 54 years) experience a mental or substance abuse disorder. The most common mental illnesses in the workplace are alcohol abuse or dependence (9% of workers); major depression (8%); and social anxiety disorder (7%). Most importantly for employees and employers is that 71 percent of workers with mental illnesses have never sought help from a medical or mental-health specialist for their symptoms.

For depression, in particular, approximately 80 percent of persons with depression reported some level of functional impairment because of their depression, and 27 percent reported serious difficulties in work and home life. The condition can also have a large effect on productivity. In a three-month period, patients with depression miss an average of 4.8 workdays and suffer 11.5 days of reduced productivity. Depression alone is estimated to cause 200 million lost workdays each year at a cost to employers of $17 to $44 billion.

Employers and employees have, in turn, had to bear the burden of rising healthcare costs. There has been a 97 percent increase in premiums for employer-sponsored health coverage since 2002. Most of the financial burden of mental-health disorders are not from the cost to treat the illness. It is because of income loss from unemployment, expenses for social support, and indirect costs—such as workers' compensation, short- and long-term disability, presenteeism (the measurable extent to which health symptoms, conditions, and diseases adversely affect the work productivity of individuals who choose to remain at work) and absenteeism.

Complications because of untreated chronic diseases and mental-health disorders are the primary cause of missed work and increased presenteeism. Even though there has been increased attention to mental health in recent years, social stigma and discrimination associated with mental illnesses remain a significant barrier to an individual's health and employment. These issues often affect whether or not an individual will apply for a job or promotion when qualified. Stigma and discrimination may also prevent an employee from seeking help contributing to presenteeism and absenteeism and if treatment is sought out it may complicate the transition back to work. Both managers and coworkers alike are often unaware or uncertain about how to interact with someone recovering from a mental-health disorder.

Many employees will not voluntarily disclose that they suffer from a chronic disease or mental-health disorder for fear of being stigmatized. This burden leads to added stress that can exacerbate their condition. In addition, not divulging this information prevents the employer from understanding to what extent some of these health issues are problems and subsequently taking action, such as changing the work environment through a workplace health program.

For example, some instances of this include how organizing and structuring work can contribute to job-related stress that can put the individual at an increased risk for chronic diseases such as cardiovascular disease. These organizational stressors include psychosocial stressors such as high job demands, low job control for the worker, or social isolation; scheduling issues including shift work or long hours; the physical demands of work whether the position is mostly sedentary or involves heavy physical exertion; exposure to hazardous chemicals such as tobacco smoke or lead; and the broader work environmental conditions (e.g., noise, heat, cold, little access to healthy food).

Through a workplace health program, employers can identify and take steps to improve the work environment to minimize the effect these organizational factors have on employee physical and mental health.

SCOPE FOR IMPROVEMENT

Although both chronic disease and mental-health disorders are common, strategies exist that can prevent or effectively treat the conditions. Modifiable risk behaviors (i.e., tobacco use, physical inactivity, and poor nutrition) that contribute to a number of chronic diseases and mental-health disorders can be targeted and a point of emphasis of a workplace health program. It is never too late to address both modifiable individual risk factors and environmental risk factors such as job stressors. For those that need treatment for more serious disease, the benefits component of a comprehensive workplace health program can provide access to professional therapy, medications, self-help, and community support programs.

What are the Best Practices for Maintaining Employees' Mental Health and Chronic Disease Status?

The Substance Abuse and Mental Health Services Administration have developed a tool kit to help workplaces become more mental-health-friendly. It describes program and practice strategies that address overall well-being by placing emphasis on both physical and mental health. The main elements of a mental-health-friendly workplace include:

- A workforce where diversity is valued
- Healthcare that treats mental illnesses with the same urgency as physical illnesses
- Programs and practices that promote and support employee health-wellness and work–life balance
- Training for managers and supervisors in mental health workplace issues, including identifying problems and processes for referral and evaluation

- Protections for the confidentiality of employee health information
- An Employee Assistance Program (EAP) or other appropriate referral resources to assist managers and employees
- Support for employees who seek treatment or who require hospitalization such as disability leave and planning for a return to work
- Regular communication and education to all employees regarding health and wellness, and similar topics that promote a climate of acceptance that reduces stigma and discrimination in the workplace

Successful programs take a comprehensive approach to health. A comprehensive program includes education, early detection and screening, program integration, and changes to the work environment to encourage healthy behaviors. The example below shows how both employers and employees can take steps to prevent and reduce work-related stress.

Establishing a workplace culture that recognizes employees for their good work, values each individual, requires that management actions are consistent with company values, and provides career development opportunities for employees, enhances employee self-confidence and productivity. Offering stress-reduction classes and employee options such as physical activity programs improve employees' physical and emotional resiliency and help them recognize and manage their own stress responses. Stress is better tolerated when employees protect their overall health through healthy behaviors such as physical activity.

The EAPs can play a critical role in reducing individual employee stress related to family caregiving or other work–life balance issues. The EAPs are designed to offer confidential short-term counseling and information to employees for work and personal concerns that may affect workplace performance. These programs may be in-house or contracted services for counseling, education, and referral. The EAPs may include information on child and elder-care services, support groups, stress reduction classes, alcohol and substance misuse treatment, mental health including depression, marital counseling, management consultation, and a variety of other important topics for managers and employees. The EAPs provide support for all levels of employees from the front line to management personnel and often for employee family members as well.

Employers can use various policy approaches that can decrease the stress effects of shiftwork and long work hours such as interference with family life through organizational change. The number of time workers spends with family and friends depends on the flexibility of their work schedule and other social and leisure time commitments. Employers can consider several strategies to design work schedules to improve work-life balance, worker satisfaction, and productivity. There is currently a limited amount of knowledge and research regarding shift work schedules and these strategies are only suggestions. It is important to remember that alterations to shift schedules affect all aspects of work and home life, so caution should be exercised when considering these strategies including planning some free weekends, examining start and end times, and keeping the schedule regular and predictable.

SUCCESS STORY

The Copenhagen healthy bus project (1999 to 2004) was an action research project that introduced more than 200 interventions to improve the health, well-being, and work environment of more than 3,000 Danish bus drivers in the greater Copenhagen area. Drivers have consistently been shown to be at increased risk of heart disease, hypertension, cancer, and job stress due in part to the lack of control drivers have over their routes, schedules, and daily traffic. Because of the combination of physical and mental health risk factors found among this group of workers, researchers decided to test comprehensive interventions that would focus on four main domains:

1. Lifestyle
2. Psychosocial factors (i.e., occupational stress)
3. Physical work environment
4. How work was organized in a large-scale intervention study

One of the main project goals was to identify how employers could influence job function and how to help companies provide the kinds of support that would reduce stress and chronic diseases.

A key component of the design of the interventions was in building relationships and trust among stakeholders. These included the driver and their union representatives, employers, and Copenhagen Traffic, that are responsible for the overall management of public bus services. Initially, they all viewed health in terms of individual responsibility and tied primarily to lifestyle. Over time the concepts of how physical health, mental health, and the organizational work environment influence overall health moved the stakeholders into a stage of readiness to change the poor health outcomes among drivers that had persisted for 50 years and addressed comprehensively many health issues that are related at multiple levels—both individually and organizationally.

Worksite health interventions included:

- Testing more flexible work schedules
- Better communication between management and drivers
- Smoking cessation program
- Nutrition courses
- Providing fresh fruit in each garage
- Educating managers in personnel management and communication
- Self-defense course
- "Know your bus" physical work environment
- More resources for bus preventive maintenance
- Joint labor-management meetings

Section 39.2 | Mental-Health Conditions in the Workplace: Your Legal Rights

This section includes text excerpted from "Depression, PTSD, and Other Mental-Health Conditions in the Workplace: Your Legal Rights," U.S. Equal Employment Opportunity Commission (EEOC), December 12, 2016. Reviewed October 2019.

If you have depression, posttraumatic stress disorder (PTSD), or other mental-health condition, you are protected against discrimination and harassment at work because of your condition, you have workplace privacy rights, and you may have a legal right to get reasonable accommodations that can help you perform and keep your job. The following, briefly explain these rights, which are provided by the Americans with Disabilities Act (ADA). You may also have additional rights under other laws, such as the Family and Medical Leave Act (FMLA) and various medical insurance laws.

IS MY EMPLOYER ALLOWED TO FIRE ME BECAUSE I HAVE A MENTAL-HEALTH CONDITION?

No. It is illegal for an employer to discriminate against you simply because you have a mental-health condition. This includes firing you, rejecting you for a job or promotion, or forcing you to take leave.

An employer does not have to hire or keep people in jobs they cannot perform, or employ people who pose a "direct threat" to safety (a significant risk of substantial harm to self or others). But an employer cannot rely on myths or stereotypes about your mental-health condition when deciding whether you can perform a job or whether you pose a safety risk. Before an employer can reject you for a job based on your condition, it must have objective evidence that you cannot perform your job duties, or that you would create a significant safety risk, even with reasonable accommodation.

AM I ALLOWED TO KEEP MY CONDITION PRIVATE?

In most situations, you can keep your condition private. An employer is only allowed to ask medical questions (including questions about mental health) in four situations:

- When you ask for a reasonable accommodation
- After it has made you a job offer, but before employment begins, as long as everyone entering the same job category is asked the same questions
- When it is engaging in affirmative action for people with disabilities (such as an employer tracking the disability status of its applicant pool in order to assess its recruitment and hiring efforts, or a public sector employer considering whether special hiring rules may apply), in which case you may choose whether to respond

- On the job, when there is objective evidence that you may be unable to do your job or that you may pose a safety risk because of your condition

You also may need to discuss your condition to establish eligibility for benefits under other laws, such as the FMLA. If you do talk about your condition, the employer cannot discriminate against you, and it must keep the information confidential, even from coworkers. If you wish to discuss your condition with coworkers, you may choose to do so.

WHAT IF MY MENTAL-HEALTH CONDITION COULD AFFECT MY JOB PERFORMANCE?

You may have a legal right to a reasonable accommodation that would help you do your job. A reasonable accommodation is some type of change in the way things are normally done at work. Just a few examples of possible accommodations include altered break and work schedules (e.g., scheduling work around therapy appointments), quiet office space or devices that create a quiet work environment, changes in supervisory methods (e.g., written instructions from a supervisor who usually does not provide them), specific shift assignments, and permission to work from home.

You can get a reasonable accommodation for any mental-health condition that would, if left untreated, "substantially limit" your ability to concentrate, interact with others, communicate, eat, sleep, care for yourself, regulate your thoughts or emotions, or do any other "major life activity." (You do not need to actually stop treatment to get the accommodation.)

Your condition does not need to be permanent or severe to be "substantially limiting." It may qualify by, for example, making activities more difficult, uncomfortable, or time-consuming to perform compared to the way that most people perform them. If your symptoms come and go, what matters is how limiting they would be when the symptoms are present. Mental-health conditions, such as major depression, PTSD, bipolar disorder, schizophrenia, and obsessive-compulsive disorder (OCD) should easily qualify, and many others will qualify as well.

HOW CAN I GET A REASONABLE ACCOMMODATION?

Ask for one. Tell a supervisor, human resources (HR) manager, or other appropriate people that you need a change at work because of a medical condition. You may ask for an accommodation at any time. Because an employer does not have to excuse poor job performance, even if it was caused by a medical condition or the side effects of medication, it is generally better to get a reasonable accommodation before any problems occur or become worse. (Many people choose to wait to ask for accommodation until after they receive a job offer, however, because it is very hard to prove illegal discrimination that takes place before a job offer). You do not need to have a particular accommodation in mind, but you can ask for something specific.

WHAT WILL HAPPEN AFTER I ASK FOR A REASONABLE ACCOMMODATION?

Your employer may ask you to put your request in writing and to generally describe your condition and how it affects your work. The employer also may ask you to submit a letter from your healthcare provider documenting that you have a mental-health condition and that you need an accommodation because of it. If you do not want the employer to know your specific diagnosis, it may be enough to provide documentation that describes your condition more generally (by stating, for example, that you have an "anxiety disorder"). Your employer also might ask your healthcare provider whether particular accommodations would meet your needs. You can help your healthcare provider understand the law of reasonable accommodation.

If a reasonable accommodation would help you to do your job, your employer must give you one unless the accommodation involves significant difficulty or expense. If more than one accommodation would work, the employer can choose which one to give you. Your employer cannot legally fire you or refuse to hire or promote you, because you asked for a reasonable accommodation or because you need one. It also cannot charge you for the cost of the accommodation.

WHAT IF THERE IS NO WAY I CAN DO MY REGULAR JOB, EVEN WITH AN ACCOMMODATION?

If you cannot perform all the essential functions of your job to normal standards and have no paid leave available, you still may be entitled to unpaid leave as a reasonable accommodation if that leave will help you get to a point where you can perform those functions. You may also qualify for leave under the FMLA, which is enforced by the U.S. Department of Labor (DOL).

If you are permanently unable to do your regular job, you may ask your employer to reassign you to a job that you can do as a reasonable accommodation, if one is available.

WHAT IF I AM BEING HARASSED BECAUSE OF MY CONDITION?

Harassment based on a disability is not allowed under the ADA. You should tell your employer about any harassment if you want the employer to stop the problem. Follow your employer's reporting procedures if there are any. If you report the harassment, your employer is legally required to take action to prevent it from occurring in the future.

WHAT SHOULD I DO IF I THINK THAT MY RIGHTS HAVE BEEN VIOLATED?

The U.S. Equal Employment Opportunity Commission (EEOC) can help you decide what to do next, and conduct an investigation if you decide to file a charge of discrimination. Because you must file a charge within 180 days of the alleged violation in order to take further legal action (or 300 days if the employer is also covered by a state or local employment discrimination law), it is best to begin the process early. It is illegal for your employer to retaliate against you for contacting the EEOC or filing a charge.

Chapter 40 | Legal Requirements to Qualify for Social Security Disability Benefits

To qualify for Social Security disability benefits, you must first have worked in jobs covered by Social Security. Then you must have a medical condition that meets Social Security's definition of disability. In general, a monthly benefit is paid to people who are unable to work for a year or more because of a disability.

Benefits usually continue until you are able to work again on a regular basis. There are also a number of special rules, called "work incentives," that provide continued benefits and healthcare coverage to help you make the transition back to work.

If you are receiving Social Security disability benefits when you reach full retirement age, your disability benefits automatically convert to retirement benefits, but the amount remains the same.

HOW MUCH WORK DO YOU NEED?

In addition to meeting our definition of disability, you must have worked long enough—and recently enough—under Social Security to qualify for disability benefits.

This chapter contains text excerpted from the following sources: Text in this chapter begins with excerpts from "Benefits Planner: Disability—How You Qualify," U.S. Social Security Administration (SSA), June 27, 2018; Text under the heading "Disability Evaluation under Social Security" is excerpted from "Disability Evaluation under Social Security," U.S. Social Security Administration (SSA), February 1, 2001. Reviewed October 2019; Text under the heading "Which Mental Disorders Are Evaluate under Each Listing Category?" is excerpted from "12.00 Mental Disorders—Adult," U.S. Social Security Administration (SSA), January 24, 2006. Reviewed October 2019.

Social Security work credits are based on your total yearly wages or self-employment income. You can earn up to four credits each year.

The amount needed for work credit changes from year to year. In 2019, for example, you earn one credit for each $1,360 in wages or self-employment income. When you have earned $5,440, you have earned your four credits for the year.

The number of work credits you need to qualify for disability benefits depends on your age when you become a person with a disability. Generally, you need 40 credits, 20 of which were earned in the last 10 years ending with the year you become a person with a disability. However, younger workers may qualify with fewer credits.

WHAT IS MEANT BY DISABILITY?

The definition of disability under social security is different than other programs. Social security pays only for total disability. No benefits are payable for partial disability or for short-term disability.

You are considered a person with a disability under Social security rules if:

- You cannot do the work that you did before
- It is decided that you cannot adjust to other work because of your medical condition(s)
- Your disability has lasted or is expected to last for at least one year or to result in death

This is a strict definition of disability. Social security program rules assume that working families have access to other resources to provide support during periods of short-term disabilities, including workers' compensation, insurance, savings, and investments.

HOW IS IT DECIDED IF YOU ARE A PERSON WITH A DISABILITY?

If you have enough work to qualify for disability benefits, a step-by-step process is used involving five questions. They are:

1. Are You Working?

If you are working in 2019 and your earnings average more than $1,220 a month, you generally cannot be considered a person with a disability.

If you are not working, your application will be sent to the Disability Determination Services (DDS) office that will make the decision about your medical condition. The DDS uses Steps two to five below to make the decision.

2. Is Your Condition "Severe"?

Your condition must significantly limit your ability to do basic work, such as lifting, standing, walking, sitting, and remembering—for at least 12 months. If it does not, it will be decided that you are not a person with a disability.

If your condition does interfere with basic work-related activities, step three is followed.

3. Is Your Condition Found in the List of Disabling Conditions?

For each of the major body systems, a list of medical conditions that are considered so severe that it prevents a person from completing a substantial gainful activity is maintained. If your condition is not on the list, it is up to the DDS to decide if it is as severe as a medical condition that is on the list. If it is, it is decided that you are a person with a disability. If it is not, then step four is carried out.

4. Can You Do the Work You Did Previously?

At this step, it is decided if your medical impairment(s) prevents you from performing any of your past work. If it does not, it is decided you do not have a qualifying disability. If it does, then step five is done.

5. Can You Do Any Other Type of Work?

If you cannot do the work you did in the past, it is checked if there is other work you can do despite your impairment(s).

Your medical conditions and your age, education, past work experience, and any transferable skills you may have are all considered. If you cannot do other work, it is decided that you are a person with a disability. If you can do other work, it will be decided that you do not have a qualifying disability and your claim will be denied.

SPECIAL SITUATIONS

Most people who receive disability benefits are workers who qualify on their own records and meet the work and disability requirements described. However, there are some situations you may not know about:

- If you are visually impaired or have low vision
- If you are the worker's widow or widower
- Benefits for a child with a disability
- Benefits for wounded warriors and veterans

SPECIAL RULES FOR PEOPLE WHO ARE VISUALLY IMPAIRED OR HAVE LOW VISION

You are considered to be legally visually impaired under Social Security rules if your vision cannot be corrected to better than 20/200 in your better eye or if your visual field is 20 degrees or less, even with a corrective lens. Many people who meet the legal definition of visual impairment still have some sight and may be able to read large print and get around without a cane or a guide dog.

If you do not meet the legal definition of visual impairment, you may still qualify for disability benefits if your vision problems alone or combined with other health problems prevent you from working.

There are a number of special rules for people who are visually impaired that recognize the severe impact of visual impairment on a person's ability to work. For example, the monthly earnings limit for people who are visually impaired is generally higher than the limit that applies to a person without a disability.

In 2019, the monthly earnings limit is $2,040.

BENEFITS FOR WIDOWS OR WIDOWERS WITH A DISABILITY

If something happens to a worker, benefits may be payable to their widow, widower, or surviving divorced spouse with a disability if the following conditions are met:

- She or he is between ages 50 and 60
- Their condition meets the definition of disability for adults
- The disability started before or within seven years of the worker's death

Widows, widowers, and surviving divorced spouses cannot apply online for survivors' benefits. However, if they want to apply for benefits, they should contact Social Security immediately at 800-772-1213 to request an appointment. (If they are hard of hearing, they should call our toll-free TTY number at 800-325-0778).

If they are a person with a disability, they can speed up the application process if they complete an Adult Disability Report and have it available at the time of their appointment.

BENEFITS FOR A CHILD WITH A DISABILITY

A child under age 18 may be a person with a disability, but it is not required to consider the child's disability when deciding if she or he qualifies for benefits as your dependent. The child's benefits normally stop at age 18 unless she or he is a full-time student in an elementary or high school (benefits can continue until age 19) or is a person with a disability.

Adults with a Disability before Age 22

An adult with a disability before age 22 may be eligible for child's benefits if a parent is deceased or starts receiving retirement or disability benefits. It is considered a "child's" benefit because it is paid on a parent's Social Security earnings record.

The "adult child"—including an adopted child, or, in some cases, a step-child, grandchild, or step-grandchild—must be unmarried, age 18 or older, have a disability that started before age 22, and meets the definition of disability for adults.

It is not necessary that the adult child ever worked. Benefits are paid based on the parent's earnings record.

- An adult child must not have substantial earnings. The number of earnings considered "substantial" increases each year. In 2019, this means working and earning more than $1,220 a month.

What If the Adult Child Is Already Receiving SSI Benefits or Disability Benefits on Her or His Own Record?

An adult child already receiving SSI benefits or disability benefits on her or his own record should still check to see if benefits may be payable on a parent's earnings record. Higher benefits might be payable and entitlement to Medicare may be possible.

How Is It Decided If an Adult "Child" Is Disabled for SSDI Benefits?

If a child is age 18 or older, her or his disability is evaluated the same way as the disability for any adult. The application is sent to the Disability Determination Services in your state that completes the disability decision.

What Happens If the Adult Child Gets Married

If she or he receives benefits as an adult with a disability since childhood, the benefits generally end if she or he gets married. However, some marriages (for example, to another adult a child has a disability) are considered protected.

The rules vary depending on the situation. Contact a Social Security representative at 800-772-1213 (If you are hard of hearing, call the toll-free TTY number at 800-325-0778) to find out if the benefits can continue.

If they are a person with a disability, they can speed up the application process if they complete an Adult Disability Report and have it available at the time of their appointment.

DISABILITY EVALUATION UNDER SOCIAL SECURITY

Disability evaluation under Social Security has been specially prepared to provide physicians and other health professionals with an understanding of the disability programs administered by the Social Security Administration (SSA). It explains how each program works, and the kinds of information a health professional can furnish to help ensure sound and prompt determinations and decisions on disability claims.

The listings are just part of how it is decided if a person is disabled. For adults, the past work experience is also considered, the severity of medical conditions, age, education, and work skills.

Disability Determination Process

Most Social Security disability claims are initially processed through a network of local SSA field offices and state agencies (usually called

"Disability Determination Services" or "DDSs"). Subsequent appeals of unfavorable determinations may be decided in a DDS or by an administrative law judge in SSA's Office of Hearing Operations.

Social Security Disability Planner for Applying for Disability Benefits Online

Social Security representatives in the field offices usually obtain applications for disability benefits in person, by telephone, by mail, or by filing online. The application and related forms ask for a description of the claimant's impairment(s), treatment sources, and other information that relates to the alleged disability. The "claimant" is the person who is requesting disability benefits.

The field office is responsible for verifying nonmedical eligibility requirements, which may include age, employment, marital status, or Social Security coverage information. The field office then sends the case to a DDS for evaluation of disability.

The DDSs, which are fully funded by the federal government, are State agencies responsible for developing medical evidence and rendering the initial determination on whether or not a claimant is a person with a disability or visually impaired under the law.

Usually, the DDS tries to obtain evidence from the claimant's own medical sources first. If that evidence is unavailable or insufficient to make a determination, the DDS will arrange for a consultative examination (CE) to obtain the additional information needed. The claimant's treating source is the preferred source for the CE, but the DDS may obtain the CE from an independent source. After completing its development of the evidence, trained staff at the DDS makes the initial disability determination.

Then, the DDS returns the case to the field office for appropriate action. If the DDS found that a claimant is a person with a disability, SSA completes any outstanding nondisability development, computes the benefit amount, and begins paying benefits. If the claimant was found not to be a person with a disability, the file is kept in the field office in case the claimant decides to appeal the determination.

WHICH MENTAL DISORDERS ARE EVALUATED UNDER EACH LISTING CATEGORY?

1. Neurocognitive Disorders

- These disorders are characterized by a clinically significant decline in cognitive functioning. Symptoms and signs may include, but are not limited to, disturbances in memory, executive functioning (that is, higher-level cognitive processes; for example, regulating attention, planning, inhibiting responses, decision-making), visual-spatial functioning, language and speech, perception, insight, judgment, and insensitivity to social standards.
- Examples of disorders that are evaluated in this category include major neurocognitive disorder; dementia of the Alzheimer type; vascular dementia; dementia due to a medical condition, such as a metabolic disease (for example, late-onset Tay-Sachs disease), human immunodeficiency virus infection, vascular malformation, progressive brain tumor, neurological disease (for example, multiple sclerosis, Parkinsonian syndrome, Huntington disease), or traumatic brain injury; or substance-induced cognitive disorder associated with drugs of abuse, medications, or toxins.
- This category does not include the mental disorders that are evaluated under intellectual disorder, autism spectrum disorder, and neurodevelopmental disorders.

2. Schizophrenia Spectrum and Other Psychotic Disorders

- These disorders are characterized by delusions, hallucinations, disorganized speech, or grossly disorganized or catatonic behavior, causing a clinically significant decline in functioning. Symptoms and signs may include, but are not limited to, inability to initiate and persist in goal-directed activities, social withdrawal, flat or inappropriate affect, poverty of thought and speech, loss of interest or pleasure, disturbances of mood, odd beliefs and mannerisms, and paranoia.
- Examples of disorders that are evaluated in this category include schizophrenia, schizoaffective disorder, delusional

disorder, and psychotic disorder due to another medical condition.

3. Depressive, Bipolar, and Related Disorders

- These disorders are characterized by an irritable, depressed, elevated, or expansive mood, or by a loss of interest or pleasure in all or almost all activities, causing a clinically significant decline in functioning. Symptoms and signs may include, but are not limited to, feelings of hopelessness or guilt, suicidal ideation, a clinically significant change in body weight or appetite, sleep disturbances, an increase or decrease in energy, psychomotor abnormalities, disturbed concentration, pressured speech, grandiosity, reduced impulse control, sadness, euphoria, and social withdrawal.
- Examples of disorders that are evaluated in this category include bipolar disorder (I or II), cyclothymic disorder, major depressive disorder, persistent depressive disorder (dysthymia), and bipolar or depressive disorder due to another medical condition.

4. Intellectual Disorder

- This disorder is characterized by significantly subaverage general intellectual functioning, significant deficits in current adaptive functioning, and the manifestation of the disorder before age 22. Signs may include, but are not limited to, poor conceptual, social, or practical skills evident in your adaptive functioning.
- The disorder that is evaluated in this category may be described in the evidence as an intellectual disability, an intellectual developmental disorder.
- This category does not include the mental disorders that are evaluated under neurocognitive disorders, autism spectrum disorder, or neurodevelopmental disorders.

5. Anxiety and Obsessive-Compulsive Disorders

- These disorders are characterized by excessive anxiety, worry, apprehension, and fear, or by avoidance of feelings, thoughts, activities, objects, places, or people. Symptoms and signs may include, but are not limited to, restlessness, difficulty concentrating, hyper-vigilance, muscle tension, sleep disturbance, fatigue, panic attacks, obsessions and compulsions, constant thoughts and fears about safety, and frequent physical complaints.

- Examples of disorders that are evaluated in this category include social anxiety disorder, panic disorder, generalized anxiety disorder, agoraphobia, and obsessive-compulsive disorder.
- This category does not include the mental disorders that are evaluated under trauma and stressor-related disorders.

6. Somatic Symptom and Related Disorders

- These disorders are characterized by physical symptoms or deficits that are not intentionally produced or feigned, and that, following a clinical investigation, cannot be fully explained by a general medical condition, another mental disorder, the direct effects of a substance, or a culturally sanctioned behavior or experience. These disorders may also be characterized by a preoccupation with having or acquiring a serious medical condition that has not been identified or diagnosed. Symptoms and signs may include, but are not limited to, pain and other abnormalities of sensation, gastrointestinal symptoms, fatigue, a high level of anxiety about personal health status, abnormal motor movement, pseudoseizures, and pseudo-neurological symptoms, such as visual impairment or a person who is hard of hearing.
- Examples of disorders that are evaluated in this category include somatic symptom disorder, illness anxiety disorder, and conversion disorder.

7. Personality and Impulse-Control Disorders

- These disorders are characterized by enduring, inflexible, maladaptive, and pervasive patterns of behavior. Onset typically occurs in adolescence or young adulthood. Symptoms and signs may include, but are not limited to, patterns of distrust, suspiciousness, and odd beliefs; social detachment, discomfort, or avoidance; hypersensitivity to negative evaluation; an excessive need to be taken care of; difficulty making independent decisions; a preoccupation with orderliness, perfectionism, and control; and inappropriate, intense, impulsive anger and behavioral expression grossly out of proportion to any external provocation or psychosocial stressors.

- Examples of disorders that are evaluated in this category include paranoid, schizoid, schizotypal, borderline, avoidant, dependent, obsessive-compulsive personality disorders, and intermittent explosive disorder.

8. Autism Spectrum Disorder

- These disorders are characterized by qualitative deficits in the development of reciprocal social interaction, verbal and nonverbal communication skills, and symbolic or imaginative activity; restricted repetitive and stereotyped patterns of behavior, interests, and activities; and stagnation of development or loss of acquired skills early in life. Symptoms and signs may include, but are not limited to, abnormalities and unevenness in the development of cognitive skills; unusual responses to sensory stimuli; and behavioral difficulties, including hyperactivity, short attention span, impulsivity, aggressiveness, or self-injurious actions.
- Examples of disorders that are evaluated in this category include autism spectrum disorder with or without accompanying intellectual impairment and autism spectrum disorder with or without accompanying language impairment.
- This category does not include the mental disorders that are evaluated under neurocognitive disorders, intellectual disorder, and neurodevelopmental disorders.

9. Neurodevelopmental Disorders

- These disorders are characterized by onset during the developmental period, that is, during childhood or adolescence, although sometimes they are not diagnosed until adulthood. Symptoms and signs may include, but are not limited to, underlying abnormalities in cognitive processing (for example, deficits in learning and applying verbal or nonverbal information, visual perception, memory, or a combination of these); deficits in attention or impulse control; low frustration tolerance; excessive or poorly planned motor activity; difficulty with organizing (time, space, materials, or tasks); repeated accidental injury; and deficits in social skills. Symptoms and signs specific to tic disorders include sudden, rapid, recurrent, nonrhythmic, motor movement or vocalization.
- Examples of disorders that are evaluated in this category include specific learning disorder, borderline intellectual functioning, and tic disorders (such as Tourette syndrome).
- This category does not include the mental disorders that are evaluated under neurocognitive disorders, autism spectrum disorder, or personality and impulse-control disorders.

10. Eating Disorders

- These disorders are characterized by disturbances in eating behavior and preoccupation with, and excessive self-evaluation of, body weight and shape. Symptoms and signs may include, but are not limited to, restriction of energy consumption when compared with individual requirements; recurrent episodes of binge eating or behavior intended to prevent weight gain, such as self-induced vomiting, excessive exercise, or misuse of laxatives; mood disturbances, social withdrawal, or irritability; amenorrhea; dental problems; abnormal laboratory findings; and cardiac abnormalities.
- Examples of disorders that are evaluated in this category include anorexia nervosa, bulimia nervosa, binge-eating disorder, and avoidant/restrictive food disorder.

11. Trauma and Stressor-Related Disorders

- These disorders are characterized by experiencing or witnessing a traumatic or stressful event, or learning of a traumatic event occurring to a close family member or close friend, and the psychological aftermath of clinically significant effects on functioning. Symptoms and signs may include, but are not limited to, distressing memories, dreams, and flashbacks related to the trauma or stressor; avoidant behavior; diminished interest or participation in significant activities; persistent negative emotional states (for example, fear, anger) or persistent inability to experience positive emotions (for example, satisfaction, affection); anxiety; irritability; aggression; exaggerated startle response; difficulty concentrating; and sleep disturbance.
- Examples of disorders that are evaluated in this category include posttraumatic stress disorder and other specified trauma, and stressor-related disorders (such as adjustment-like disorders with prolonged duration without the prolonged duration of stressor).
- This category does not include the mental disorders that are evaluated under anxiety and obsessive-compulsive disorders, and cognitive impairments that result from neurological disorders, such as a traumatic brain injury, which are evaluated under neurocognitive disorders.

Chapter 41 | Mental-Health Coverage under the Affordable Care Act

The Affordable Care Act (ACA) provides one of the largest expansions of mental-health and substance-use disorder (SUD) coverage in a generation. Beginning in 2014 under the law, all new small group and individual market plans were required to cover 10 Essential Health Benefit categories, including mental-health and substance-use disorder services, and required to cover them at parity with medical and surgical benefits. The ACA builds on the Paul Wellstone and Pete Domenici Mental Health Parity and Addiction Equity Act of 2008 (MHPAEA, or the federal parity law), which requires group health plans and insurers that offer mental-health and substance-use disorder benefits to provide coverage that is comparable to coverage for general medical and surgical care.

While almost all large group plans and most small group plans include coverage for some mental-health and substance-use disorder services, there are gaps in coverage and many people with some coverage of these services do not currently receive the benefit of federal parity protections. The final rule implementing the Essential Health Benefits (EHBs) directed nongrandfathered health plans in the individual and small group markets to cover mental-health and substance-use disorder services as well as to comply with the federal parity law requirements beginning in 2014.

This chapter includes text excerpted from "Affordable Care Act Will Expand Mental Health and Substance-Use Disorder Benefits and Parity Protections for 62 Million Americans," Office of the Assistant Secretary for Planning and Evaluation (ASPE), February 2013. Reviewed October 2019.

MENTAL-HEALTH AND SUBSTANCE-USE DISORDER BENEFITS PRIOR TO THE AFFORDABLE CARE ACT

About one-third of those who were currently covered in the individual market have no coverage for substance-use disorder services and nearly 20 percent have no coverage for mental-health services, including outpatient therapy visits and inpatient crisis intervention and stabilization. In addition, even when individual market plans provided these benefits, the federal parity law did not apply to these plans to ensure that coverage for mental-health and substance-use disorder services was generally comparable to coverage for medical and surgical care.

In the small group market, coverage of mental-health and substance-use disorder treatment was more common than in the individual market. It is estimated that about 95 percent of those with small group market coverage had substance abuse and mental-health benefits. Again, the federal parity law did not apply to small group plans. In many states, state parity laws offer those covered in this market some parity protection, but most state parity laws are narrower than the federal parity requirement.

In addition, 47.5 million Americans lacked health insurance coverage altogether, and 25 percent of uninsured adults have a mental-health condition or substance-use disorder, or both.

THE AFFORDABLE CARE ACT: BETTER COVERAGE FOR MENTAL-HEALTH AND SUBSTANCE-USE DISORDERS

The ACA and its implementing regulations, building on the MHPAEA, expanded coverage of mental-health and substance-use disorder benefits and federal parity protections in three distinct ways:

1. By including mental-health and substance-use disorder benefits in the EHBs
2. By applying federal parity protections to mental-health and substance-use disorder benefits in the individual and small group markets
3. By providing more Americans with access to quality healthcare that includes coverage for mental-health and substance-use disorder services

Essential Health Benefits

First, under the statute, treatment for mental-health and substance-use disorders is a benefit category covered as part of the package of EHBs available to all Americans in nongrandfathered plans in the individual and small group markets as of January 1, 2014. The EHBs final rule, released in 2014, ensures that consumers purchasing insurance can be confident that their health plan will provide the care they need if they get sick. Including mental-health and substance-use disorder treatment in this package means

- About 3.9 million people who were currently covered in the individual market gained either mental-health or substance-use disorder coverage, or both
- Also, an estimated 1.2 million individuals who were currently in small group plans were able to receive mental-health and substance-use disorder benefits under the ACA

Parity in the Individual and Small Group Markets

Second, the U.S. Department of Health and Human Services (HHS) finalized regulations that applied federal parity rules to mental-health and substance-use disorder benefits included in EHBs. As a result, Americans accessing coverage through nongrandfathered plans in the individual and small group markets were able to count on mental-health and substance-use disorder coverage that is comparable to their general medical and surgical coverage.

- Under this approach, 7.1 million Americans who were currently covered in the individual market and who currently had some mental-health and substance-use disorder benefits would have access to coverage of EHBs that conforms to federal parity protections as provided for under the ACA and the MHPAEA.
- In addition, because the application of parity to EHBs also applied to those currently enrolled in nongrandfathered plans in the small group market, 23.3 million current enrollees in small group plans also received the benefit of having mental-health and substance-use disorder benefits that are subject to the federal parity law.

Table 41.1. Essential Health Benefits Provisions of the Affordable Care Act

	Individuals who will gain mental-health, substance-use disorder, or both benefits under the Affordable Care Act, including federal parity protections	**Individuals with existing mental-health and substance-use disorder benefits who will benefit from federal parity protections**	**Total individuals who will benefit from federal parity protections as a result of the Affordable Care Act**
Individuals currently in individual plans	3.9 million	7.1 million	11 million
Individuals currently in small group plans	1.2 million	23.3 million	24.5 million
Individuals currently uninsured	27 million	n/a	27 million
Total	32.1 million	30.4 million	62.5 million

NOTE: These estimates include individuals and families who are currently enrolled in grandfathered coverage. Grandfathered plans are not required to comply with the Essential Health Benefits provisions of the ACA.

Increasing Access to Quality Healthcare

Finally, the ACA expanded insurance coverage to a projected 27 million previously uninsured Americans through access to private health insurance in the individual and small group markets, the marketplaces, and Medicaid. EHBs, including mental-health and substance-use disorder services subject to parity requirements, and made available to this newly covered population.

In total, through the ACA, 32.1 million Americans gained access to coverage that includes mental-health and/or substance-use disorder benefits that comply with federal parity requirements and an additional 30.4 million Americans who currently had some mental-health and substance-abuse benefits were able to benefit from the federal parity protections. By building on the structure of the MHPAEA, the ACA extended federal parity protections to a projected 62 million Americans.

Chapter 42 | Mental-Health Rehabilitation Programs for Veterans

PROGRAM DESCRIPTION

Mental Health Residential Rehabilitation Treatment Programs (MH RRTPs) (including Domiciliary and RRTPs) provide residential rehabilitative and clinical care to veterans who have a wide range of problems, illnesses, or rehabilitative care needs which may include mental-health and substance-use disorders (SUDs), co-occurring medical conditions and psychosocial needs such as homelessness and unemployment. All of these programs provide a 24/7 therapeutic setting utilizing both professional and peer supports. Treatment focuses on the veteran's needs, abilities, strengths, and preferences.

There are several types of programs which include the following:

Domiciliary Residential Rehabilitation Treatment Programs

A Domiciliary Residential Rehabilitation Treatment Programs (DRRTP) provides a residential level of care for veterans with issues related to medical, mental-health, substance-use disorders, posttraumatic stress disorders (PTSD), and homelessness. These programs are larger residential programs with multiple units serving various veteran populations based on need.

Domiciliary Care for Homeless Veterans

A Domiciliary Care for Homeless Veterans (DCHV) provides a residential level of care for a homeless veteran population. A DCHV may be a standalone program or a unit within a larger DRRTP.

This chapter includes text excerpted from "Mental Health Residential Rehabilitation Treatment Programs," Benefits.gov, USA.gov, July 18, 2013. Reviewed October 2019.

Health Maintenance Domiciliary

Health maintenance domiciliary beds provide a residential level of care for veterans. Health maintenance domiciliary programs focus on symptom reduction and stabilization as part of the rehabilitative approach to facilitating community integration. A health maintenance domiciliary may be a standalone unit or part of a larger DRRTP.

General Domiciliary (General Dom) or Psychosocial Residential Rehabilitation Treatment Programs

These programs provide a residential treatment level of care for a general veteran population with a variety of needs. General Dom beds are a part of a larger DRRTP while Psychosocial Residential Rehabilitation Treatment Programs (PRRTPs) are standalone units.

Domiciliary Posttraumatic Stress Disorder or Posttraumatic Stress Disorder Residential Rehabilitation Treatment Program

These programs provide the residential level of care to veterans with posttraumatic stress disorder including the provision of services for veterans who have experienced military sexual trauma (MST). Domiciliary posttraumatic stress disorder (Dom PTSD) may be part of a larger DRRTP while a Posttraumatic Stress Disorder Residential Rehabilitation Treatment Program (PTSD-RRTP) is a standalone unit.

Domiciliary Substance Abuse or Substance Abuse Residential Rehabilitation Treatment Program

These programs provide a residential level of care to veterans with substance-use disorders. Dom substance abuse (Dom SA) beds may be part of a larger DRRTP while a Substance Abuse Residential Rehabilitation Treatment Program (SARRTP) is a standalone program.

Compensated Work Therapy-Transitional Residence

General Compensated Work Therapy-Transitional Residence (CWT-TR) offers therapeutic work-based residential rehabilitation services designed to facilitate successful community reintegration for veterans. The program does not target any particular mental-health diagnosis. The program requires concurrent enrollment in the Compensated Work Therapy program.

PROGRAM REQUIREMENTS

You must be enrolled in the U.S. Department of Veterans Affairs (VA) healthcare system (or qualify based on one of the exceptions in the law).

U.S. Department of Veterans Affairs

Generally, in order to receive VA benefits and services the veteran or servicemember's character of discharge or service must be under other than dishonorable conditions (e.g., honorable, under honorable conditions, general). However, individuals receiving undesirable, bad conduct, and other types of dishonorable discharges may qualify for VA benefits depending on a determination made by VA.

In addition to basic eligibility criteria for care in the VA healthcare system, the veteran must:

- Be assessed as not meeting the criteria for acute psychiatric or medical admission
- Have tried a less restrictive treatment alternative, or one was unavailable
- Be assessed as requiring the structure and support of a residential treatment environment
- Be assessed as not a significant risk of harm to self or others
- Be lacking a stable lifestyle or living arrangement that is conducive to recovery
- Be capable of self-preservation and basic self-care
- Have identified treatment and rehabilitation needs, which can be met by the program

If the veteran's circumstance cannot be accommodated by the program, alternative services must be considered within the medical centers, Veterans integrated service networks (VISNs), or Veterans health administration's (VHA's) mental-health continuum of care and appropriate alternate treatment arrangements made.

A single screening determines whether a veteran is appropriate for admission to any of the facility's MH RRTPs. To facilitate access, screenings are conducted on all normal business days. Given the comorbid disorders typical of a veteran being screened for residential services, consideration needs to be given to which MH RRTP provides the "best" fit, rather than the ideal match.

Domiciliary Care has some eligibility rules of its own. You must meet one of these criteria:

- Your annual income must not exceed the maximum annual Improved Disability VA Pension Rate or
- VA must determine that you have no adequate means of support

You can find the special eligibility rules for Domiciliary Residential Rehabilitation and Treatment (Domiciliary Care) in the Code of Federal Regulations (CFR). Here are the references: Title 38, CFR 17.46, 17.47, and 17.48.

Chapter 43 | Disability Rights Movement

Treatment and perceptions of disability have undergone transformation since the 1900s. This has happened largely because people with disabilities have demanded and created those changes. Like other civil rights movements, the disability rights movement has a long history. Examples of activism can be found among various disability groups dating back to the 1800s. Many events, laws, and people have shaped this development. To date, the 1990 Americans with Disabilities Act (ADA) and the subsequent ADA Amendments Act (2008) are the movement's greatest legal achievements. The ADA is a major civil-rights law that prohibits discrimination of people with disabilities in many aspects of public life. The disability rights movement continues to work hard for equal rights.

Organizations by and for people with disabilities have existed since the 1800s. However, they exploded in popularity in the 1900s. The League of the Physically Handicapped organized in the 1930s, fighting for employment during the Great Depression. In the 1940s a group of psychiatric patients came together to form "We Are Not Alone." They supported patients in the transition from hospital to the community. In 1950, several local groups came together and formed the National Association for Retarded Children (NARC). By 1960, NARC had tens of thousands of members, most of whom were parents. They were dedicated to finding alternative forms of care and education for their children. Meanwhile, people with disabilities received assistance through the leadership of various presidents in the 1900s. President Truman formed the National Institute of Mental Health (NIMH) in 1948. Between the years 1960 and 1963, President Kennedy organized several planning committees to treat and research disability.

This chapter includes text excerpted from "Disability History: The Disability Rights Movement," National Park Service (NPS), U.S. Department of the Interior (DOI), December 1, 2017.

The U.S. Congress has passed many laws that support disability rights either directly or by recognizing and enforcing civil rights. Civil rights laws such as Brown versus Board of Education and its decision that school segregation is unconstitutional laid the groundwork for recognizing the rights of people with disabilities. Several sections of the 1973 Rehabilitation Act, which specifically address disability discrimination, are especially important to the disability rights movement. Section 501 supports people with disabilities in the federal workplace and in any organization receiving federal tax dollars. Section 503 requires affirmative action, which supports employment and education for members of traditionally disadvantaged minority groups. Section 504 prohibits discrimination against individuals with disabilities in the workplace and in their programs and activities. Section 508 guarantees equal or comparable access to technological information and data for people with disabilities. The regulations for Section 504 of the Rehabilitation Act of 1973 were written but not implemented. In 1977, the disability rights community was tired of waiting and demanded that President Carter sign the regulations. Instead, a task force was appointed to review them. Afraid that the review would weaken the protections of the Act, the American Coalition of Citizens with Disabilities (ACCD) insisted they be enacted as written by April 5, 1977, or the coalition would take action. When the date arrived and the regulations remained unsigned, people across the country protested by sitting-in in federal offices of Health, Education, and Welfare (the agency responsible for the review). In San Francisco, the sit-in at the federal building lasted until April 28, when the regulations were finally signed, unchanged. This was, according to organizer Kitty Cone, the first time that "disability really was looked at as an issue of civil rights rather than an issue of charity and rehabilitation at best, pity at worst."

The 1975 Education of All Handicapped Children Act guaranteed children with disabilities the right to public school education. These laws have occurred largely due to the concerted efforts of disability activists protesting for their rights and working with the federal government. In all, the United States Congress passed more than 50 pieces of legislation between the 1960s and the passage of the ADA in 1990.

Self-advocacy groups have also shaped the national conversation around disability. Self-advocacy means representing one's own interests. Such groups include DREDF (Disability Rights Education and Defense Fund), ADAPT (Americans Disabled for Accessible Public Transportation, later changed to Americans Disabled Attendant Programs Today), and the CIL (Centers for Independent Living). The CIL provides services for people with disabilities in the community. The CIL began in the early 1960s at Cowell Memorial Hospital. Located in California, Cowell Memorial Hospital was once listed on the National Register of Historic Places (NRHP). The building is now demolished, but its legacy remains. The hospital supported the "Rolling Quads" and the "Disabled Students Program" at the University of California Berkeley. Students Ed Roberts and John Hessler founded both organizations. Both men lived with physical disabilities and needed to find housing options after their acceptance to the university. University dormitories could not manage Roberts' iron lung, an assistive breathing device for people with polio, or Hessler's physical needs. Hessler and Roberts instead lived at Cowell Memorial Hospital when they arrived at college in the early 1960s. With the assistance of the College of San Mateo counselor Jean Wirth, they demanded access to the school and encouraged other students with physical disabilities to attend UC Berkeley. They also influenced school architecture and planning. UC Berkeley eventually created housing accommodations for these students. It was there that the students planted the seed of the independent living movement. The independent living movement supports the idea that people with disabilities can make their own decisions about living, working, and interacting with the surrounding community. This movement is a reaction to centuries of assisted living, psychiatric hospitals, and doctors and parents who had made decisions for individuals with disabilities.

Roberts, Hessler, Wirth, and others established the Disabled Students Program at UC Berkeley. Although this was not the first program of its kind, Illinois offered similar services beginning in the 1940s, the UC Berkeley Program was groundbreaking. They promoted inclusion for all kinds of students on campus. The program inspired universities across the country to create similar organizations. Many of these organizations are still active today.

The Rolling Quads and CIL are among the two groups from the disability rights movement. Disability activists also work with other communities to attain their goals. People form communities based on shared values, ideas, and identity. The strength and activism of a community can help change attitudes across society at large. Perceptions of disability and resulting treatment often intersect with other groups advocating for their civil and human rights. One example of this change is the treatment of the Lesbian Gay Bisexual Transgender Queer (LGBTQ) community. Doctors regarded homosexuality as a disease well into the 20th century. They could send men and women to psychiatric hospitals for their sexual preference. It was not until the 1970s that this "diagnosis" changed.

The Dr. Franklin Kameny Residence is part of this important history. Kameny had served as an astronomer and worked with the U.S. Army Map Service. In the 1950s, he refused to reveal his sexual orientation to the government. In response, the U.S. government fired Kameny from his job. Kameny spent the rest of his life working as an activist and advocate for LGBTQ rights. His home provided the space for people to safely express and identify themselves. In 1973, Kameny successfully led the fight to abolish homosexuality from the American Psychiatric Association's (APA) Diagnostic and Statistical Manual of Mental Disorders (DSM). The DSM is the official handbook used by healthcare professionals to diagnose psychiatric issues and disabilities. This decision legally removed the status of homosexuality as a disorder. It also helped shift perceptions of homosexuality. More and more people began to understand it was not wrong or defective. The Kameny Residence continues to help us recognize and embrace the work of the gay civil rights community.

Other activists also took to the streets and demonstrated for disability rights. Some of these protests occurred at locations that are today listed on the NRHP. In 1988, students at Gallaudet University, the only American university specifically for hard to hear students, led the "Deaf President Now" protest. Students made several demands, calling for a Deaf president and majority Deaf population on the Board of Trustees. This week-long protest resulted successfully in the appointment of the president, Dr. I. King Jordan. Their protest inspired inclusion and integration across communities.

Two years later in 1990, protesters gathered on the steps of the United States Capitol building. They were anxiously awaiting the passage of the ADA, which had stalled due to issues around transportation. Public transit companies fought against the strict regulations for accessibility, and their lobbying efforts slowed the entire process. In response, a group of individuals with disabilities headed for the Capitol. They tossed aside their wheelchairs, walkers, and crutches and ascended the steps. This event has since become known as the "Capitol Crawl." By dragging themselves up the stairs, these protesters expressed their daily struggles due to physical barriers. In so doing, they highlighted the need for accessibility. Iconic images of this event spread across the country. The ADA ultimately passed in July 1990 and was signed by President George H.W. Bush. The ADA and other civil rights legislation have transformed opportunities for people with disabilities. However, over 25 years later, there is still much work to be done.

Chapter 44 | Neurodiversity Movement

The term "neurodiversity" combines the words "neurological" and "diversity" to create a new word that captures the reality that human brains function in a variety of ways. This term—and the intention behind it—further recognizes that these differences in brain function and behavior are just that: differences along a wide spectrum of possible functions and behaviors. The term "normal" was once used to characterize people with no known neurological disorders (the so-called neuro-typical), but the neurodiversity movement reminds us that using the term "normal" in this manner is inaccurate, because any of these variations are normal and naturally occurring variations in the human genome. Judy Singer, the Australian social scientist on the autism spectrum who coined the term, further points out that neurological differences across humanity are comparable to variations that occur naturally in plants and animals in biodiversity.

Refocusing the lens through which people view neurological function allows us, at both the individual and societal level, to see each other as people first as we shift away from a cultural lens than sees some of us as abnormal or defined primarily by one particular variety of neurological functioning.

DIFFERENCE, NOT DEFICIENCY

The neurodiversity movement continues to shift societal attitudes about and perceptions of people with neurological disorders, including attention deficit/hyperactivity disorder (ADHD), dyspraxia, dyslexia, autism/autism spectrum disorders, and Tourette syndrome. These shifts in attitudes also affect how medical researchers, healthcare providers, and individuals react when they encounter unexpected behaviors in others. One problematic cultural reaction in such moments is social discomfort and one previously common cultural assumption is that the person with a neurological disability is somehow "behaving badly." While these assumptions remain common among some people, it is useful to remember that many neurological disorders are invisible at first glance.

Recognizing that neurological functioning exists on a spectrum encourages healthcare providers, medical researchers, readers, and society at large to remember that people with a disability, any disability, may be "differently abled" than the neuro-typical, but their particular kind of neurological functioning may actually enhance their abilities in some areas. Refocusing the lens through which a disabled person is viewed also serves as a useful reminder that each of us is endeavoring to live a full, productive, and healthy life, and each desires and deserves to be recognized as someone whose life is of tremendous value.

Shifting Our Cultural Lens

In cultural terms, the concept of neurodiversity reminds us that the specific physiological features of and restrictions experienced by a person with a disability do not equate with that person being "abnormal," "deficit," or in need of "fixing," as cultural stereotyping might suggest, but rather defines a person with a neurological disability as someone whose abilities differ from those of the majority of people who do not have a neurological disability. Recognizing this distinction can enrich our personal interactions while welcoming people of all neurological functions into our communities, which will likewise result in a drop in social stigmas that do real harm to people with disabilities.

The neurodiversity movement further amplifies the reality that, while social stereotyping may define a person with a disability as being unhealthy or someone with a poor quality of life, the actual quality of life of a person with a disability may not be lacking at all or may only be lacking because specific and addressable cultural and environmental barriers restrict their ability to engage fully in the same daily activities that neuro-typical members of society enjoy.

Functional Inclusion

Recognizing that "disability" is what occurs when a person's functional needs have not been addressed in his or her physical and social environments also reminds us to recognize and address physical and environmental challenges that all people—including those with a disability—experience to some degree because of our unique human traits. And recognizing that such barriers prevent people from participating fully in society further reminds us that such participation barriers are not the result of any personal deficit or shortcoming.

Technological advances and shifts in our social understanding of disability are helping to eliminate participation barriers so that all people can be supported and enabled to live full and independent lives to the best of their abilities. Adjusting our cultural lens also reminds us that we all have a social responsibility to ensure that we create and sustain accessible environments and communities in which each of us is supported, valued, and enabled to live our best lives.

Cultural Inclusion

As mentioned previously, Judy Singer makes the point that neurological differences across humanity are comparable to variations that occur naturally in plants and animals. Members of the neurodiversity civil-rights movement point out that homosexuality was deemed to be a psychiatric disorder until the late 1980s, but the idea of "curing" homosexuality is now generally recognized as a stigmatizing and harmful attempt to harm people whose sexual attractions merely differ from the majority of the population.

Some members of the neurodiversity movement, including the vocal "autistic and proud" community, also assert that attempts to "cure" their conditions is systematic discrimination practiced by an "ableist" society that continues to marginalize and oppress neuro-diverse people.

The Anti-Cure Movement

One branch of the neurodiversity movement, in fact, considers any effort to "cure" neurological difference as comparable to eugenics and consider such attempts to do so to be on par with genocide.

Ironically, this view further stigmatizes people with neurological disabilities who wish to be cured from, say, from self-harming autistic behaviors such as head-banging, or from the incontinence that some people with autism experience. This branch of the movement deems such people to be self-haters and equates their hope for a cure with the "internalized homophobia" experienced by some members of the stigmatized homosexual population.

Others point out that the end goal of any medical intervention is to improve the overall quality of life of a person with a disability (or other medical disorder) and that developing treatments that enable people to live their lives more fully is neither motivated by politics nor stigma, but rather an effort to help everyone live better and more independent lives.

Examining the particular voices of this diverse movement offers us an opportunity to engage in meaningful debate if we remember that each of us wishes to be seen as capable and whole just as we are instead of being defined as someone who needs to be "fixed."

References

1. Robison, John Elder. "What Is Neurodiversity?" *Psychology Today*, October 7, 2013.
2. Clements, Thomas. "The Problem with the Neurodiversity Movement," Quillette, October 15, 2017.

Part 5 | **Additional Resources**

Chapter 45 | Organizations That Provide Services for People with Mental Disabilities

GOVERNMENT AGENCIES THAT PROVIDE INFORMATION ABOUT MENTAL DISABILITIES

Administration for Community Living (ACL)
330 C. St., S.W.
Washington, DC 20201
Phone: 202-401-4634
Website: www.acl.gov
E-mail: aclinfo@acl.hhs.gov

Americans with Disabilities Act (ADA)
Toll-Free: 800-514-0301
Toll-Free TTY: 800-514-0383
Website: www.ada.gov

Benefits.gov
Website: www.benefits.gov

Centers for Disease Control and Prevention (CDC)
1600 Clifton Rd.
Atlanta, GA 30329-4027
Toll-Free TTY: 888-232-6348
Website: www.cdc.gov

Clearinghouse on Disability Information (CODI)
Office of Special Education and Rehabilitative Services (OSERS), U.S. Department of Education (ED)
550 12th St., S.W.
Rm. 5133
Washington, DC 20202-2550
Phone: 202-245-7307
TTD: 202-205-5637
Fax: 202-245-7636
Website: www2.ed.gov/about/offices/list/osers/codi.html

Resources in this chapter were compiled from several sources deemed reliable; all contact information was verified and updated in October 2019.

***Eunice Kennedy Shriver* National Institute of Child Health and Human Development (NICHD)**
Information Resource Center (IRC)
P.O. Box 3006
Rockville, MD 20847
Toll-Free: 800-370-2943
Toll-Free Fax: 866-760-5947
Website: www.nichd.nih.gov
E-mail: NICHDInformation ResourceCenter@mail.nih.gov

Genetic and Rare Diseases Information Center (GARD)
P.O. Box 8126
Gaithersburg, MD 20898-8126
Toll-Free: 888-205-2311
Toll-Free TTY: 888-205-3223
Fax: 301-251-4911
Website: rarediseases.info.nih.gov
E-mail: gardinfo@nih.gov

girlshealth.gov
Office on Women's Health (OWH)
200 Independence Ave., S.W.
Rm. 712E
Washington, DC 20201
Toll-Free: 800-994-9662
Website: www.girlshealth.gov

HealthCare.gov
Centers for Medicare & Medicaid Services (CMS)
Toll-Free: 800-318-2596
Toll-Free TTY: 855-889-4325
Website: www.healthcare.gov

Internal Revenue Service (IRS)
Joint Board for the Enrollment of Actuaries (JBEA)
1111 Constitution Ave., N.W.
SE:RPO, Rm. 3422
Washington, DC 20224
Toll-Free: 800-829-1040
Toll-Free TTY/TDD: 800-829-4059
Website: www.irs.gov
E-mail: nhqjbea@irs.gov

National Council on Disability (NCD)
1331 F. St., N.W., Ste. 850
Washington, DC 20004
Phone: 202-272-2004
Fax: 202-272-2022
Website: www.ncd.gov
E-mail: ncd@ncd.gov

National Heart, Lung, and Blood Institute (NHLBI)
Center for Health Information
P.O. Box 30105
Bethesda, MD 20824-0105
Phone: 301-592-8573
Website: www.nhlbi.nih.gov
E-mail: nhlbiinfo@nhlbi.nih.gov

National Highway Traffic Safety Administration (NHTSA)
1200 New Jersey Ave., S.E.
W. Bldg.
Washington, DC 20590
Toll-Free: 888-327-4236
Phone: 202-366-4000
Toll-Free TTY: 800-424-9153
Website: www.nhtsa.gov

National Institute of Mental Health (NIMH)
Office of Science Policy, Planning, and Communications (OSPPC)
6001 Executive Blvd.
Rm. 6200, MSC 9663
Bethesda, MD 20892-9663
Toll-Free: 866-615-NIMH (866-615-6464)
TTY: 301-443-8431
Toll-Free TTY: 866-415-8051
Fax: 301-443-4279
Website: www.nimh.nih.gov
E-mail: nimhinfo@nih.gov

National Institute of Neurological Disorders and Stroke (NINDS)
NIH Neurological Institute
P.O. Box 5801
Bethesda, MD 20824
Toll-Free: 800-352-9424
Website: www.ninds.nih.gov

National Institute on Aging (NIA)
Bldg. 31, Rm. 5C27
31 Center Dr., MSC 2292
Bethesda, MD 20892
Toll-Free: 800-222-2225
Toll-Free TTY: 800-222-4225
Website: www.nia.nih.gov
E-mail: niaic@nia.nih.gov

National Institute on Deafness and Other Communication Disorders (NIDCD)
Office of Health Communication and Public Liaison (OCPL)
31 Center Dr., MSC 2320
Bethesda, MD 20892-2320
Toll-Free: 800-241-1044
Phone: 301-827-8183
Toll-Free TTY: 800-241-1055
Website: www.nidcd.nih.gov
E-mail: nidcdinfo@nidcd.nih.gov

National Institute on Disability, Independent Living, and Rehabilitation Research (NIDILRR)
330 C. St., S.W., Rm. 1304
Washington, DC 20201
Phone: 202-795-7398
Fax: 202-205-0392
Website: acl.gov/about-acl/about-national-institute-disability-independent-living-and-rehabilitation-research
E-mail: nidilrr-mailbox@acl.hhs.gov

National Institute on Drug Abuse (NIDA)
Office of Science Policy and Communications (OSPC)
6001 Executive Blvd.
Rm. 5213, MSC 9561
Bethesda, MD 20892
Phone: 301-443-1124
Website: www.drugabuse.gov

National Institute on Drug Abuse (NIDA) for Teens
Public Information and Liaison Branch (PILB)
Phone: 301-443-1124
Website: teens.drugabuse.gov

National Institutes of Health (NIH)
9000 Rockville Pike
Bethesda, MD 20892
Phone: 301-496-4000
TTY: 301-402-9612
Website: www.nih.gov

Office of Disability Employment Policy (ODEP)
U.S. Department of Labor (DOL)
200 Constitution Ave., N.W.
Washington, DC 20210
Toll-Free: 866-ODEP-DOL (866-633-7365)
Phone: 202-693-7880
Website: www.dol.gov/odep
E-mail: odep@dol.gov

Office of Disease Prevention and Health Promotion (ODPHP)
Office of the Assistant Secretary for Health (OASH), Office of the Secretary
1101 Wootton Pkwy
Ste. LL100
Rockville, MD 20852
Fax: 240-453-8281
Website: health.gov
E-mail: odphpinfo@hhs.gov

Office of the Assistant Secretary for Planning and Evaluation (ASPE)
U.S. Department of Health and Human Services (HHS)
200 Independence Ave., S.W.
Rm. 415F
Washington, DC 20201
Phone: 202-690-7858
Website: aspe.hhs.gov

Office of the Assistant Secretary for Preparedness and Response (ASPR)
U.S. Department of Health and Human Services (HHS)
200 Independence Ave., S.W.
Rm. 638G
Washington, DC 20201
Website: www.phe.gov

Office on Women's Health (OWH)
U.S. Department of Health and Human Services (HHS)
200 Independence Ave., S.W.
Rm. 712E
Washington, DC 20201
Toll-Free: 800-994-9662
Phone: 202-690-7650
Fax: 202-205-2631
Website: www.womenshealth.gov

Substance Abuse and Mental Health Services Administration (SAMHSA)
5600 Fishers Ln.
Rockville, MD 20857
Toll-Free: 877-SAMHSA-7 (877-726-4727)
Toll-Free TTY: 800-487-4889
Website: www.samhsa.gov
E-mail: SAMHSAInfo@samhsa.hhs.gov

U.S. Commission on Civil Rights (USCCR)
1331 Pennsylvania Ave., N.W.
Ste. 1150
Washington, DC 20425
Phone: 202-376-7700
TTY: 202-376-8116
Website: www.usccr.gov

U.S. Department of Education (ED)
400 Maryland Ave., S.W.
Washington, DC 20202
Toll-Free: 800-USA-LEARN (800-872-5327)
Website: www2.ed.gov

U.S. Department of Health and Human Services (HHS)
Hubert H. Humphrey Bldg.
200 Independence Ave., S.W.
Washington, DC 20201
Toll-Free: 877-696-6775
Website: www.hhs.gov

U.S. Department of Justice (DOJ)
950 Pennsylvania Ave., N.W.
Washington, DC 20530-0001
Phone: 202-514-2000
Toll-Free TTY/TDD: 800-877-8339
Website: www.justice.gov

U.S. Department of Labor (DOL)
200 Constitution Ave., N.W.
Washington, DC 20210
Toll-Free: 866-4-USA-DOL (866-487-2365)
Toll-Free TTY: 877-889-5627
Website: www.dol.gov

U.S. Department of the Interior (DOI)
1849 C. St., N.W.
Washington, DC 20240
Phone: 202-208-3100
Website: www.doi.gov
E-mail: feedback@ios.doi.gov

U.S. Department of Transportation (DOT)
1200 New Jersey Ave., S.E.
Washington, DC 20590
Toll-Free: 855-368-4200
Phone: 202-366-4000
Website: www.transportation.gov

U.S. Department of Veterans Affairs (VA)
810 Vermont Ave., N.W.
Washington, DC 20420
Toll-Free: 844-698-2311
TTY: 711-698-2311
Website: www.va.gov

U.S. Equal Employment Opportunity Commission (EEOC)
Toll-Free: 800-669-4000
Toll-Free TTY: 800-669-6820
Website: www.eeoc.gov
E-mail: info@eeoc.gov

U.S. Social Security Administration (SSA)
Office of Public Inquiries and Communications Support (OPICS)
1100 W. High Rise
6401 Security Blvd.
Baltimore, MD 21235
Toll-Free: 800-772-1213
Toll-Free TTY: 800-325-0778
Website: www.ssa.gov

USA.gov
Toll-Free: 844-USA-GOV1 (844-872-4681)
Website: www.usa.gov

PRIVATE AGENCIES THAT PROVIDE INFORMATION ABOUT MENTAL DISABILITIES

ADvancing States
241 18th St., S., Ste. 403
Arlington, VA 22202
Phone: 202-898-2578
Fax: 202-898-2583
Website: www.advancingstates.org
E-mail: info@advancingstates.org.

AMA Insurance Agency, Inc.
330 N. Wabash Ave., Ste. 39300
Chicago, IL 60611-5885
Toll-Free: 888-627-5883
Toll-Free Fax: 877-588-7488
Website: www.amainsure.com
E-mail: wecare@amainsure.com

American Association of People with Disabilities (AAPD)
2013 H. St., N.W.
Fifth Fl.
Washington, DC 20006
Toll-Free: 800-840-8844
Phone: 202-521-4316
Website: www.aapd.com
E-mail: communications@aapd.com

American Psychiatric Association Foundation (APA Foundation)
800 Maine Ave., S.W.
Ste. 900
Washington, DC 20024
Toll-Free: 888-35PSYCH (888-357-7924)
Phone: 202-559-3888
Website: www.apafdn.org
E-mail: apafoundation@psych.org

Association of University Centers on Disabilities (AUCD)
1100 Wayne Ave.
Ste. 1000
Silver Spring, MD 20910
Phone: 301-588-8252
Fax: 301-588-2842
Website: www.aucd.org
E-mail: aucdinfo@aucd.org

Bacharach Institute for Rehabilitation
61 W. Jimmie Leeds Rd.
Pomona, NJ 08240
Phone: 609-652-7000
Fax: 609-748-5427
Website: www.bacharach.org
E-mail: email@bacharach.org

Be The Match®
National Marrow Donor Program® (NMDP)
500 N. Fifth St.
Minneapolis, MN 55401-1206
Toll-Free: 800-MARROW2 (800-627-7692)
Website: bethematch.org

Center on Technology and Disability (CTD)
FHI 360
1825 Connecticut Ave., N.W.
Washington, DC 20009
Website: www.ctdinstitute.org
E-mail: ctd@fhi360.org

Disabilities, Opportunities, Internetworking, and Technology (DO-IT)
University of Washington (UW)
P.O. Box 354842
Seattle, WA 98195-4842
Toll-Free: 888-972-DOIT (888-972-3648)
Phone: 206-685-DOIT (206-685-3648)
TTY: 509-328-9331
Fax: 206-221-4171
Website: www.washington.edu/doit
E-mail: doit@uw.edu

Disability:IN
3000 Potomac Ave.
Alexandria, VA 22305
Website: disabilityin.org
E-mail: info@disabilityIN.org

ERIC Clearinghouse on Disabilities and Gifted Education (ERIC EC)
Council for Exceptional Children (CEC)
1920 Association Dr.
Reston, VA 20191
Toll-Free: 800-328-0272
Website: www.icdri.org/Education/eric.htm
E-mail: ericec@cec.sped.org

Federation for Children with Special Needs (FCSN)
529 Main St.
Ste. 1M3
Boston, MA 02129
Toll-Free: 800-331-0688
Phone: 617-236-7210
Fax: 617-241-0330
Website: fcsn.org
E-mail: fcsninfo@fcsn.org

Indiana Institute on Disability and Community (IIDC)
1905 N. Range Rd.
Bloomington, IN 47408-9801
Phone: 812-855-6508
Fax: 812-855-9630
Website: www.iidc.indiana.edu/pages/about
E-mail: iidc@indiana.edu

Learning Disabilities Association of America (LDA)
P.O. Box 10369
Pittsburgh, PA 15234-1349
Phone: 412-341-1515
Fax: 412-344-0224
Website: www.ldaamerica.org
E-mail: info@ldaamerica.org

Learning Disabilities Worldwide (LDW)
179 Bear Hill Rd., Ste. 104
Waltham, MA 02451
Phone: 978-897-5399
Website: www.ldworldwide.org
E-mail: help@ldworldwide.org

National Aging and Disability Transportation Center (NADTC)
Toll-Free: 866-983-3222
Website: www.nadtc.org
E-mail: contact@nadtc.org

National Center for Learning Disabilities (NCLD)
One Thomas Cir., N.W.
Ste. 700
Washington, DC 20005
Phone: 212-545-7510
Website: www.ncld.org
E-mail: info@ncld.org

National Center on Health, Physical Activity and Disability (NCHPAD)
4000 Ridgeway Dr.
Birmingham, AL 35209
Toll-Free: 800-900-8086
Fax: 205-313-7475
Website: www.nchpad.org
E-mail: email@nchpad.org

National Council on Independent Living (NCIL)
2013 H. St., N.W.
Sixth Fl.
Washington, DC 20006
Toll-Free: 844-778-7961
Phone: 202-207-0334
TTY: 202-207-0340
Fax: 202-207-0341
Website: www.ncil.org
E-mail: ncil@ncil.org

National Disability Rights Network (NDRN)
820 First St., N.E.
Ste. 740
Washington, DC 20002
Phone: 202-408-9514
TDD/TTY: 202-408-9521
Fax: 202-408-9520
Website: www.ndrn.org
E-mail: info@ndrn.org

National Organization on Disability (NOD)
77 Water St., Ste. 204
New York, NY 10005
Phone: 646-505-1191
Fax: 646-505-1184
Website: www.nod.org
E-mail: info@nod.org

Pan American Health Organization (PAHO)
525 23rd St., N.W.
Washington, DC 20037
Phone: 202-974-3000
Fax: 202-974-3663
Website: www.paho.org

Paralyzed Veterans of America (PVA)
801 18th St., N.W.
Washington, DC 20006-3517
Toll-Free: 800-424-8200
Toll-Free TTY: 800-795-4327
Website: pva.org
E-mail: info@pva.org

Rehabilitation International (RI Global)
866 United Nations Plaza
Office 422
New York, NY 10017
Phone: 212-420-1500
Fax: 212-505-0871
Website: www.riglobal.org
E-mail: info@riglobal.org

SEMO Alliance for Disability Independence, Inc. (SADI)
755 S. Kingshighway
Cape Girardeau, MO 63701
Toll-Free: 800-898-7234
Phone: 573-651-6464
Fax: 573-651-6565
Website: www.sadi.org

Smart Kids with Learning Disabilities®, Inc. (SKLD)
38 Kings Hwy., N.
Westport, CT 06880
Website: www.smartkidswithld.org

TASH
1101 15th St., N.W.
Ste. 1212
Washington, DC 20005
Phone: 202-467-5730
Fax: 202-540-9019
Website: tash.org
E-mail: info@tash.org

Tourette Association of America Inc. (TAA)
42-40 Bell Blvd.
Ste. 205
Bayside, NY 11361
Toll-Free: 888-4-TOURET (888-486-8738)
Website: tourette.org
E-mail: support@tourette.org

United Cerebral Palsy Alliance (UCPA) of Hawai‘i
414 Kuwili St., Ste. 105
Honolulu, HI 96817-5362
Phone: 808-532-6744
Fax: 808-532-6747
Website: www.unitedcerebralpalsyhawaii.org
E-mail: info@unitedcerebralpalsyhawaii.org